PENGUIN BOOKS

BACK IN TEN MINUTES

Dr Mary Rintoul graduated in medicine from St Thomas's Hospital in
1961. She has spent time in general practice and is now engaged in
hospital practice. She is married to a dentist who has a long history of
intermittent back pain.

Bernard West graduated in dentistry from Sheffield University in 1969. He
was in general practice in Kent for twenty years. Like many people in his
profession, he suffered from a series of backaches and pains, and disabilities
for various periods. His attempts to devise a simpler means of coping with
these stresses brought him into contact with Mary Rintoul. After success-
fully overcoming similar problems in a wider circle of people, they agreed
to collaborate in writing *Back in Ten Minutes*, to share their knowledge of
easing poor postural pains and improving musculo-skeletal control. He has
contributed articles to professional journals and is presently working in
Health Service Management.

DR MARY RINTOUL AND BERNARD WEST

Back in Ten Minutes

AN EASY-TO-READ GUIDE AND
EXERCISE PROGRAMME TO HELP PROTECT
YOUR BACK AND IMPROVE YOUR POSTURE

PENGUIN BOOKS

PENGUIN BOOKS

Published by the Penguin Group
Penguin Books Ltd, 27 Wrights Lane, London W8 5TZ, England
Penguin Books USA Inc., 375 Hudson Street, New York, New York 10014, USA
Penguin Books Australia Ltd, Ringwood, Victoria, Australia
Penguin Books Canada Ltd, 10 Alcorn Avenue, Toronto, Ontario, Canada M4V 3B2
Penguin Books (NZ) Ltd, 182–190 Wairau Road, Auckland 10, New Zealand

Penguin Books Ltd, Registered Offices: Harmondsworth, Middlesex, England

Published in Penguin Books 1995
10 9 8 7 6 5 4 3 2 1

Typeset by Datix International Limited, Bungay, Suffolk
Filmset in 11/13 pt Monophoto Photina
Printed in England by Clays Ltd, St Ives plc

Contents

1 Back Pain – Facts and Figures

Back pain is now almost an epidemic in the West. The back is a complex structure consisting of a large number of muscles, bones, ligaments, tendons, nerves and blood-vessels and the potential for trouble is enormous. It is difficult to put accurate figures on the incidence of back pain as much of it goes unreported – many sufferers just 'grin and bear it' – but it may be helpful to give some current estimates.

- Back pain is said to be the cause of more sickness and absentee-ism than any other malady apart from colds and influenza. The cost to individual sufferers and to the country is colossal in terms of lost productivity, quite apart from the pain and misery.
- At least eighty per cent of us suffer at some time in our lives – two million-plus visit the doctor each year with back-related troubles of some sort.
- Only about ten per cent of back-pain sufferers have a specific disease or malfunction. About ninety per cent therefore show nothing seriously wrong on examination although complete agreement about diagnosis is rare.
- About forty per cent of sufferers recover within one week of the onset of back pain.
- A further twenty per cent are better within three weeks – this recovery occurs regardless of treatment given.
- A high percentage of people who have suffered an attack of back pain will have a recurrence unless remedial measures are put in hand. It is best not to attempt self-diagnosis; do go and see your doctor to eliminate any possible serious cause or condition. This may entail a specialist's opinion.

Usually the back-pain sufferer will belong to the ninety per cent who have non-specific pain. However, as far as this book is concerned, it is wise to obtain a medical all-clear first and then you can proceed with the preventive exercises. The majority of the exercises are simple and straightforward and none is strenuous.

People sometimes know themselves what gave them a bad back. It may have been any one of a myriad causes, e.g. too much gardening or DIY, lifting something heavy or awkward, doing too much sport, or not being fit enough – but often the real reason is simply that they did not treat their backs properly in daily activities. Most probably, fatigue, stress and tension all played a part.

The main problem areas of the back are:

- Lower back between the waist and buttocks.
- Upper back.
- Neck and shoulders.

Most of us have little idea how we abuse our backs in the course of our day and do not think of the damage, often unwittingly, being done. We act surprised when back pain strikes – usually unexpectedly – but we seldom take any preventive measures to counter the possibility of 'doing our back in'. Accumulated stress and strain tax the system until finally something goes wrong and a trivial movement like a hard sneeze or cough or stepping off a pavement can produce the final injury and with it a crisis of back pain.

Back pain is often the result of weak muscle tone as the back is a repository of much strain and tension. Stress from work pressures can end up lodged in the neck, shoulders or lower back and can be seen and felt in tense, taut muscles. We alter our posture to ease this discomfort and consequently it then becomes easy to throw the back out of its proper alignment. Many of us operate in a state of physical imbalance, our posture compensating unconsciously all the time in order to cope. Back pain is non-life-threatening and so has a low treatment priority at a time when NHS resources are scarce. We are required to assume more responsibility ourselves, learning how to take care of our own backs. At first, most back-pain sufferers vow to do something about their problem. After the pain has subsided, exercises are often begun in a blaze of enthusiasm but are slowly abandoned as things improve. Few people keep them up and initial good intentions are forgotten.

In fact, most back pain can be avoided with a bit of thought towards
prevention.

Many of us hold excessive muscle tension all day, without being aware of it for the most part. We have weak, tight muscles stemming from poor posture habits, gained especially at work, which are every bit as damaging, producing additional fatigue and physical stress.

Back pain can limit everyday enjoyment and interfere with our lifestyle. It can be agonizing but will almost certainly pass in time. The spine is incredibly tough and rugged – after all, it is designed to last for at least seventy years. But the old adage that a bad back puts years on you faster than anything is truer now than ever. We hope that this brief introduction has convinced you of the need to 'Do It Yourself' and learn to create your own defences against this modern-day scourge.

Warning Note

The exercises and advice given in this book are not meant for people with chronic illness or other conditions that may be affected by unsupervised exercise. Any application of the advice or recommendations following is at the reader's discretion and sole risk – it is meant for informational purposes and is not intended as a prescription. The authors strongly recommend that, prior to starting the exercises contained in this book, the reader consults his or her medical practitioner for advice and clearance to proceed.

Every care has been taken to ensure that the information contained in this book is consistent with medical opinion. It is only a guide, though, and is not meant as a substitute for your doctor's advice.

Having satisfied yourself on the above, bear in mind that there are three requirements to ensure success. These are common sense, care and commitment. You cannot do it all in one week: common sense dictates that you start gradually. All of us tend to be overenthusiastic at the start of a health regime or fitness campaign – it is easy to get carried away and possibly hurt yourself as a consequence. The care comes in doing the exercises properly, making sure that you understand what you are trying to achieve with each of them. The commitment factor comes into play when you realize that improvement is slow and steady as you work to maintain a pain-free back. No one else can do it for you – in fact, no one else is particularly interested – and it will do you a power of good to feel that you are taking responsibility for your own back.

2 About Exercise

Our aim in this book is to try and help the reader first with some general advice about exercise, and then with specific advice on exercises that will help to improve posture, protect and defend the back and, as a bonus, reduce work-induced tension and stress. We are seeking all-round postural fitness here – not training for a competitive sport.

Benefits of Exercise

Our bodies need regular exercise to function at their best.
Some benefits of exercise are:

- It can help to keep your weight down. Apart from helping you to burn calories, it tones up the muscles so that you look slimmer and feel better.
- It improves blood circulation throughout the body. Most people who have had varicose-vein operations are prescribed a strict walking schedule to speed healing.
- It keeps joints working to their full capacity and can help limit the effects of arthritis and other such degenerative diseases.
- It can aid you with an all-round decrease in tension and stress; it helps you relax and even sleep better. Exercise is even prescribed by some doctors as part of the treatment of mild depressive illnesses.

Exercise should be a part of daily life for the majority, but never too intense unless you are a serious competitor.

It is easy to get carried away by an initial burst of enthusiasm – this can be a mistake, as too much exercise can be harmful. It leads to chronic fatigue, an increased susceptibility to injury and a depressed immune system, increasing the incidence of viral infections such as colds and influenza. It is generally wise not to exercise when suffering from an infection, though this advice is usually applied to aerobic exercises such as running, cycling or serious athletic sport. A minimal daily expenditure of effort reaps great benefits. Many people feel that feverish activity is necessary when taking exercise. This is not so – in fact, low-intensity exercise is just as valuable as high-intensity exercise which can carry a large 'drop-out' factor as people become disenchanted or bored with prolonged, heavy exercise sessions after expecting quick results. 'Going for the burn' is now outdated and fast walking is regarded as more use and less harmful than excessive jogging. The idea is to treat exercise as an essential (like cleaning your teeth) and a normal part of your day. But don't go overboard – remember, we are talking about basic levels of fitness and not Olympic training.

Types of Exercise

Exercises can be grouped into three categories:

1 Aerobic
This involves building general stamina and is concerned primarily with the heart, the need for the body to take up oxygen efficiently and to work to capacity. It includes activities such as walking, running, jogging and cycling and is an essential component of an all-round exercise or fitness programme.

2 Strength
This group involves working on the muscles and muscular endurance – improving our ability to meet certain requirements of daily life with relative ease such as carrying loads, or any task needing sustained effort. We include some strength exercises in this book.

3 Flexibility (suppleness)
This involves extending our range of movement of joints and muscles and associated ligaments to enable us to bend, twist and turn as required. Flexibility is very easily lost under the rigours of daily life. Strength and flexibility are what concern us particularly regarding the protection of our backs.

6   It is general inactivity that hinders the smooth working of the

body in all its functions. It causes bones and muscles to weaken – just think how feeble a broken limb is after a few weeks in plaster. We *need* activity – to push ourselves a little – as lack of exercise means that we will almost certainly age more quickly.

Part of the problem is that most of us live in a modern, hi-tech environment with labour-saving gadgets everywhere; in our houses, gardens, offices and other workplaces. These do make life easier, and no one would advocate a return to former drudgery, but we seldom get opportunities to relieve our pent-up stress with some good hard physical exertion unless we actively seek them out. Then we may find that our bodies simply cannot cope with the increased demand. Muscles that are regularly stretched and exercised are always ready for action. Unless steps are deliberately taken, most people operate at the minimum fitness level required by a job in hand. An unfit person has far less capacity to meet a sudden call on their energy that may unexpectedly arise.

Please do not leap violently into exercise. Ease yourself gently into a routine. Try to resolve to exercise daily (we recommend some ideas and suitable combinations later) and follow through to gain the benefits. The pay-off is enormous in terms of reduced vulnerability to back pain or injury. It is true that one of the best, most effective defences against back pain (either after recovery or, better still, to prevent its occurrence) is a specific range of exercises tailored to strengthen the muscles that support and protect the back and spine.

Our best advice is to show you how to do those exercises yourself.

Warming Up

Warming up before taking any exercise is essential to avoid damage to muscles and ligaments. For our purposes, since we are not suggesting any strenuous exercises, it will also be a gentle process. Warming up acts as a pump-primer, preparing the body for action by lubricating the tissues and joints. It makes exercise easier as muscles work better when warm and relaxed. Always begin slowly – do not just leap straight into an extended stretch. Once your body gets used to the routines and adapts itself, your ability to stretch will greatly increase.

Here are a few warm-up exercises – just pick and choose to suit yourself as you get into the habit of exercising.

Spot Marching

March on the spot, gradually increasing the tempo, and lifting your knees higher. Let your arms swing back and forth.

Ceiling Stretches

(also known as the Fruit-picker's Reach). Reach up as far as you can towards the ceiling – first with one arm, then the other and finally both together. You can tilt your head back *slightly* to look at the ceiling, or else look ahead.

Arm Circles

Use large slow circles to loosen up the shoulder-joints – brush your ear as your arm circles past – first one arm, then the other and, finally, both together. Repeat in the opposite direction.

Limb Shakes

Shake one hand and arm, then the other and, finally, both together. Then do the same with your legs and feet, as swimmers do when warming up for a race.

Shoulder Rotations

Slowly rotate each shoulder first backward, then forward. Try to make each circle as big as you can manage. Keep the non-circling shoulder still. Do each shoulder in turn, then both together.

Breathing

It is always helpful to do some deep breathing. Breathe in as you swing your arms forward and up overhead, while rising up on tiptoe. Breathe out and relax as you come down.

Leg Swings

Swing each leg backward and forward while holding on to a work-top or desk for support. Gently increase the length of the swings.

Think of slowly bringing all your joints and muscles to life – 8 mobilizing and loosening them up ready for action. The goal to bear in mind is to put all your joints through a full range of movement.

Exercises to Avoid

There are some exercises that it is better not to do as they are potentially harmful.

Double Leg Raises

Avoid any exercise where you have both legs straight out and attempt to lift them off the ground at the same time. Such exercises are often recommended for the abdominal muscles but in fact the hip flexor muscles take over and this can cause greatly increased pressure in the lower back area.

Sit Ups

The same criteria apply here as in the double leg raises. The hip flexors take over early on and you get severe pulling on the lower back. Curl ups are much safer as described on page 98.

Toe Touches

This exercise involves the hamstring muscles at the back of the thighs which are often reluctant to stretch much. Toe-touching is largely achieved using the lower back muscles which are easily overstretched.

Kneeling Leg Thrusts

Most people doing this exercise lift the extended leg too high which overextends the hip-joint and compresses the lower back and intervertebral joints.

Raising Arms and Legs

When doing floor exercises, do not raise both arms and legs at the same time, again for the above reasons.

Deep Knee Bends

When doing knee bends, do not bring the knees past a right angle – in other words, keep thighs parallel to the ground. It is very easy to overstretch the knee ligaments.

Neck Rolls
Full head circles can damage the cervical vertebrae unless they are done very gently.

Points to Note
Be wary of arching your back too far as this can squeeze the spinal joints and discs. When you perform this exercise, use your hands as a support in the small of your back (see page 49).

Take care with all bending and twisting exercises, as they are potentially harmful if performed without due caution. Never stretch with locked knees – always keep the knees slightly flexed and try to bend from the hips, not the waist.

Make a commitment to regular exercise and build it up gradually. Proceed gently, use your common sense, concentrate on what you are doing and your progress will be steady and certain. And remember, there is not much point in doing all the exercises and then reverting to bad habits of slouching and slumping. Think BACK all the time.

Pelvic Tilt and Abdominal Muscles – Keys to a Strong Back

Strong abdominal muscles are an enormous benefit all round – in fact their development is crucial to achieving good posture and a strong, well-protected back. They act as a support system, working as stabilizers in movements such as bending, twisting and lifting. They help relieve stress on the lower back and support the internal organs. If they are weak, they are a major factor in lower back pain – the pelvis sags back, leading to excessive spinal curvature. This can throw the whole spine out of alignment as the upper body slumps forward.

The tighter and stronger the abdominal muscles, the more the spine and lower back area are offered support. Abdominal pressure is maintained, helping to keep the spinal curves the correct shape.

The diagram on the left on page 11 shows how strong abdominal muscles help to give good support to the spine. The diagram on the right demonstrates how weak or flabby abdominal muscles cause pressure against the front abdominal wall, draining support away from the spine. Try to think of a balloon full of air held between your two flat hands. As you squeeze one hand towards the other, you will immediately feel the pressure of the air in the balloon. This is how strong abdominal muscles help naturally to brace the spine. The key to strengthening the abdominal muscles, reducing excessive lower back slumping and supporting the spine is the **pelvic tilt** (we will abbreviate this to the PT throughout the book).

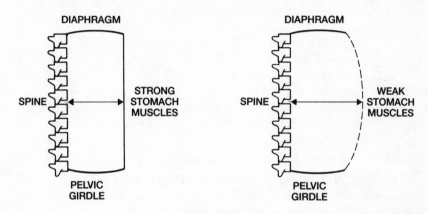

Balloon principle

As its name implies, this move controls the position of the pelvis and hence the strength and balance of the back and trunk. When you have learnt to do it, you will have a sound base upon which to develop good posture habits for all your exercises and daily activities. You will also find that standing or sitting for long periods will be far less tiring.

Pelvic Tilt – Standing

1 Stand with your back to a wall (or door) with your heels about six inches away from the wall and feet about six inches apart.
2 Allow your shoulders and buttocks to touch the wall – you should notice a gap between the small of your back and the wall where you can insert your flat hand.
3 Keep knees slightly flexed.

4 Remove your hand and then try to eliminate the gap by flattening your lower back against the wall – push it backward to make it touch the wall.
5 At the same time, look straight ahead, keep your chin level with the floor, and try to keep the back of your head against the wall. You may find this difficult at first, but in time you will be able to keep your head touching the wall as your posture improves.

It may take time to achieve this goal if you are round-shouldered, but it will be possible as you persevere and short, tight anterior shoulder muscles learn to relax and let go. Prepare to be amazed at the difference even in a short time.

Always keep your shoulders relaxed, level and down – a good tip is to remember to make the distance between your ears and shoulders as great as possible.

As you push the lower back against the wall, the pelvis will tilt upward, and this action will help smooth out excessive curvature in your lower back, as you tighten your abdominal muscles. The object of this procedure is to get the back of the head, shoulders, lower back and buttocks to touch the wall together (the lower back will not normally be in the same plane but as this is an exercise designed to tilt your pelvis, don't worry).

A tip to help you feel what you are trying to achieve is to lift one foot up on a low stool or something similar when standing against the wall so that the thigh of the raised leg is at right angles to the floor. You will immediately feel how the pelvis tilts, making it easier to get your lower back against the wall. Then, tighten your abdominal muscles and lower your foot to the ground. When you have managed to hold this position (or near), walk away from the wall trying to maintain this unaccustomed feeling of strange, but good, posture.

Practise this exercise as often as you can throughout the day until it feels more natural and less strained. It is one of the best back-defence moves you can do for yourself. Walk around holding this new position, feeling the difference. At first you will be horrified by the gap between your back and the wall, but persevere. The rapid improvement will convince you.

Pelvic Tilt – Sitting

1 Sit with your bottom as far back into the chair as you can – don't slouch.
2 Push your lower back against the back of the chair by tightening the abdominal muscles, thereby tilting your pelvis upward.
3 Keep shoulders relaxed and down – try to imagine that the top of your head is being pulled up by a string – as you do this, it will open up the chest.

As with the standing PT, a good idea is to raise one foot up on a low stool and this will help you to push your lower back against the back of the chair.

Pelvic Tilt – Lying Down

This is a useful relaxation exercise.

1 Lie on your back, arms by your sides, knees bent to about forty-five degrees, feet flat on the floor.
2 Place one hand under the small of your back, into the hollow there (as you did with the standing PT).
3 Remove your hand and get rid of the hollow by flattening the small of your back against the floor as you tighten your abdominal muscles. You will feel your hips rotating forward and your pelvis tilting upward.

The PT is the basic position in which to carry out all the exercises in this book. Try to practise this position as much as possible during the day. The spine has most protection when held in this position as its curves are in their ideal shape and are not under any strain.

3 About Posture

The spine is central to our body structure and therefore our posture, and has the following functions:

- It is the channel that houses and protects the spinal cord, which carries messages from the brain to control almost all the body's operations.
- It allows us complete flexibility and mobility.
- It acts as a framework for the body so that it can bear its own, and carry additional, weight.

The gentle S-shaped curve of a normal spine has evolved to achieve perfect weight-distribution and balance, correctly maintaining the body's centre of gravity at all times. If the back does not keep its natural S-shape for whatever reason, there is a much greater risk of pain. The position of the pelvis is also very important, as it is in relation to the pelvic girdle that the spine is grounded through the legs. Good, strong, muscle support is essential to help keep the many bones, joints, ligaments and other tissues of the spine protected and working properly. When the back muscles are in good order, they keep the spinal curves in correct relationship, leading to good posture overall. So you can understand the importance of exercise to strengthen and maintain the postural muscles as the spine bears the enormous stresses imposed upon it by daily life.

Posture Control

General Factors Involved
- The constant downward pull of gravity.
- Hereditary or genetic factors, e.g. to have one leg shorter than the other is surprisingly common and is bound to affect posture.
- Specialized, repetitive actions specific to jobs and daily routines.
- Unconscious negative habits such as stooping and slouching.

Individual Factors Involved

- Muscular strength or weakness in abdomen, back or legs.
- Hip flexibility – just watch someone who needs a hip replacement walking, and observe their gait.
- Back curve – this S-curve can be either too flat or too deep.
- Extra abdominal weight – a paunch, or pregnancy.
- Alignment of feet, knees or legs: if these are misaligned, posture is inevitably affected.
- Carriage of neck and shoulders.
- Head position in relation to the neck and shoulders – this is of prime importance in posture.

Let's take a general overview of posture.

Posture is not static but dynamic – even at rest; there are tiny imperceptible muscle movements going on all the time, even when we are asleep. Posture is a habit, a learned procedure, and can therefore be relearned if necessary. It is an unconscious behaviour pattern controlled by an automatic mechanism in any given situation, and just as conscious decisions are involved in such actions as standing, sitting, walking or carrying out specific tasks, posture habits can be altered with conscious effort. We unconsciously affect our posture in response to sudden stimuli – we stiffen up sharply or pull back our head or move instinctively without time to consider our actions.

Many of us harbour tension over the years, with the result that progressive stiffness, even lopsidedness, replace good posture. We find ourselves habitually adopting certain positions, unaware of the harm this is doing. For example, some dentists show a distinct shoulder droop on one side after years by the chair in a stooped, unnatural position. Other people in similar situations often incline their weight to one side and find that they cannot accommodate this imbalance without overusing other muscles and this adds to a normal day's fatigue.

Our posture reflects our habits. We need to learn how to respond continually to gravitational pull. Most of us take the line of least resistance; once we become used to slumping and slouching, any attempt to correct our posture feels awkward so we let it go and poor posture becomes the norm. We need to work with 15 gravity and around it, not to succumb to it. Part of the trouble is that we seldom see good posture, or follow a role model, as the postural decline starts early on in life. Good posture is striking, simply because it is rarely seen. It has lost its way from the old-fashioned concepts of bearing, deportment, or even the military ideal. Any military institution can tell you about the generally poor posture of each fresh intake of recruits.

We do not know what good posture feels like although we can recognize it when we see it. A casual glance at any crowd of people will show us how far we have fallen – and the fall is more noticeable in the Western world. The words 'poise' and 'carriage' go hand in hand with posture, conveying the image of a person standing and moving well, with balance and grace.

Posture is a major indicator of mood and generally reflects our feelings, for example the slouch of dejection or sadness, the braced neck and shoulders of the defensive. We can be stiff-necked or uptight; whatever our mood, it may be obvious to an onlooker and can influence the treatment we receive from those around us. Posture radically affects our appearance – often for the worse – and, more significantly, it almost certainly affects our physical functioning as years of misuse tire our muscle structure. Common sense should tell us that if we ignore our posture, we are much more likely to suffer from decreased vitality and even poor health.

To sum up briefly, so far: posture depends on habits – good posture stems from good habits, and the reverse is equally true. A bad posture puts the spine and back under excessive strain while a good posture relieves strain. We *can* change bad habits if we want to, and if we persevere. Poor posture can be improved dramatically. But it is not much use talking about posture unless we mean to do something about it, so we will now look at good posture and how to acquire it.

4 Good Posture – How to Achieve It

There can be no blanket description of good posture as people come in all shapes and sizes and to attempt to cover everything would be unrealistic. However, we can try to lay down a few guidelines.

An ideal posture is one where the back is subjected to the least possible strain while maintaining its normal curves: it requires a position that can be held with minimal expenditure of muscular effort and energy. That seems straightforward enough, but it is much easier to describe than it is to practise.

The real keys to good posture are first, the position of the head in relation to the spine and second, the retention of the PT which helps to keep the spinal curve in its correct alignment. Think of a string attached to the top of your head, suspended from a pulley on the ceiling and pulling you straight upward, while your chin is kept level. Don't overdo the image as the object is to regularize excessive spinal curvature but not to straighten the back entirely. Reach upward and the curves move gently back into shape. The spine and neck lengthen as the crown of the head rises towards the ceiling. Don't underestimate the importance of the position of the head. It weighs between ten and fifteen pounds and must be held correctly to help achieve a good posture.

The spine always works best when lengthened in the manner described above. Another good idea is to visualize the body as a series of boxes stacked on top of one another. If one box is pushed out somewhere, e.g. if you poke your head forward, then you will get a compensatory curve or 'box' pushed out backward.

The centre of gravity in the human frame is behind the navel, buried deep inside the abdomen when standing up normally. As you lean forward, the centre of gravity moves forward to be above your toes. You now appear, or feel to be, top-heavy, so naturally you lock your knees and tense your muscles to stop yourself falling over. Good posture means that the centre of gravity is always where it needs to be, well inside the body's parameters. This applies in any situation and is really based on common sense. It is much less tiring if the spinal curve works around the centre of gravity to help you balance; good posture is produced by this action.

Guidelines

An imaginary plumb-line dropped on the body from overhead should fall approximately through:

The ear lobe
The tip of the shoulder
The middle of the hip
Just behind the kneecap
Just in front of the ankle-bone

To get some idea of your current posture, a full-length mirror to test yourself from all angles is a great help. First of all, just stand as you normally do, observe yourself and ask some questions. For instance:

- Is your head centred squarely on your shoulders or tilted to one side – is it poked forward or pressed back and down or does it look compressed down on your neck?
- Is your spine straight or curved – are the curves excessive or flat?
- Are your shoulders level – are they rounded or held forward?
- Is your chest thrust out or sagging – is your pelvis tilted to one side – are your knees locked? Can you see tension in some muscles and slackness elsewhere?
- Is there a squashed effect from the top down – is gravity winning?

Repeat this examination from a side view – are you leaning back? After a full inspection, let it all flop and sag as if you were not aware of your posture at all. Most people get a bit of a shock as they witness the effect. Then, stand up properly using the guidelines given and feel and see the difference.

Check-list

18 1 Stand in front of the mirror.

2 See if there is anything askew that you feel you would like to change.
3 Try to put yourself in the desired new position. You may find the new position tiring at first as muscles are stretched and lengthened. This will improve as you practise and become used to the change.

To change our posture, we need to:

- Become aware of our present posture and our unconscious reactions.
- Try to improve our posture and be conscious of all our movements all the time.

Persevere with this new approach although unavoidably it will be difficult at first. You will be surprised how much you notice about yourself, probably for the first time, and what needs to be done about it. Try to be an interested spectator of your own behaviour and then practise your new-found good postural habits. So often, the advice we hear is not helpful – 'Stand up straight' or, 'Get your shoulders back' or, 'Chest out' or similar – but we still need to learn how to achieve good posture. We can all recognize it in dancers, actors and musicians and models, most of whom are taught good posture as an essential part of their training. The principles they are taught of poise – fluid, economical movement – can be applied by all of us. Few of us have natural poise – some of us require it in our jobs or professions but the rest of us must work to acquire it.

Pointers

- Stand straight – feet shoulder-width apart, weight equally on both feet.
- Keep knees slightly flexed – keep the PT.
- Shoulders should be relaxed, held back to allow the ribcage to rise. If you rotate your hands so that your palms face forward, you can actually feel your shoulders ease backward.
- Keep chin level – arms hanging loosely.
- Try to push the top of your head to the ceiling – ease the head backward at the same time.

Incidentally, the idea of practising carriage and deportment with a book or cushion on your head is a good one. Try it and see. If you bend forward with the book on your head, you can immediately feel the neck muscles tense up – they must in order to take the weight. You automatically correct your posture when you push up, to ease the strain and make the weight comfortable. This gives you an idea of the importance of head position.

Three keys to help you are:

1 Think tall – remember the pulley and the string lifting you up; keep your chin level.
2 Think broad – shoulders broad, level, relaxed – chest open.
3 Think pelvic tilt to strengthen the abdominal muscles.

Remember these points and put them into practice as often as you are able throughout the day; also remember that this increased awareness has to carry over into most aspects of your lifestyle. Get into the habit of frequent checks and take the time now and then to look at yourself.

Benefits of Good Posture

The main benefits are:

- Helps keep the spine strong and supple, using minimum energy to balance the body correctly.
- Helps the body to wear well with minimum friction and stiffness.
- When the spine is held and supported properly, the internal organs are better able to work freely.
- Good posture leads to more efficient breathing and circulation. When you stand well, your lungs can fully expand, thus helping the bellows effect and resulting in better oxygenated blood.
- When you are standing well, there is less compression of the vertebral joints and discs – you look instantly slimmer as well as regaining your full height (slouching makes you seem to lose inches).
- Not only do you look better; good posture conveys confidence. It encourages other people to respond positively to you. It reflects your attitude and even your personal competence. It has much

20

more impact than most people realize as it is one of the first things about you to strike onlookers.

- Lastly, and our main concern, it will minimize the risk of back pain.

Good posture eases tense muscles and is a key factor in repairing the damage done by a sedentary lifestyle. You are far better placed to accommodate gravity especially as you get older. It makes balance easier; physical strength is greater as you are making much better use of natural leverage. Practice does make perfect for good posture.

5 Poor Posture – Why You Should Avoid It

The detrimental effects of poor posture are not yet fully appreciated, although this is slowly changing. Even in the area of fitness, the effects of poor posture are only now coming into true focus. The causes of poor posture are so numerous that almost any reason can be given without much fear of contradiction. A large part of the problem is that we react with our body in automatic ways to certain situations or people: we have habitual responses that have become unconscious, and can be harmful as far as posture is concerned.

Much poor posture stems from poor alignment of the head with the spine. Preschool children start out well with carefree poise at play. Then the rot sets in as the child goes to school and desk work takes over, followed by homework done at a desk or table plus the normal slouching in front of the TV. The child almost invariably gets locked into a downward spiral of muscle tension and defensive positions as postural faults take over by degrees – faults which will probably become more deeply entrenched in adolescence.

As we have seen, poor posture can more easily be understood as any position where the back and associated structures are under extra or unnecessary strain. It is easy to understand how and where we impose such strain during our lives.

Environmental factors at work and during leisure too are to blame: we use poorly designed equipment – chairs, car seats, lighting, worktops – the list of possible culprits is endless. Things are changing, but there is a lot to be done yet in this field. You often hear people saying, 'My back is killing me', as they put in long hours of standing, sitting or working in awkward positions. Tension gathered during the working day emerges as back pain. We seldom notice this muscle tension arising under the stresses of a demanding job, so it is a comparatively simple matter to get subtle, harmful changes taking place. It is quite usual to favour one side of our body or the other in the course of daily activities (we may suffer Repetitive Strain Injury or RSI as a result – discussed in Chapter 7) and lack of body balance becomes normal. We develop armour in layers as we repeatedly tense up and do not deal with tension as it arises. Muscles get shortened and tight or overstretched and weak. For example, if a person spends all their time hunched over a desk, the body adapts by the rear shoulder muscles becoming longer and weaker, while the front chest and shoulder muscles become tight and short. That person is almost bound to become round-shouldered if they allow the situation to continue unchecked.

Gravity is a major player in the poor posture scenario. Weight bearing and gravity are always with us. It is easier to go with it and slouch – we can lose as much as half an inch in height during the day (this is regained at night as the body lies flat and the vertebral discs swell up again as they rehydrate and the spine regains its length – almost). Another factor is ignorance of the damage caused by poor working practices and how to change them.

Emotional factors too are to blame in certain cases. Anxiety can show itself as muscular tension especially in the neck, shoulders and back. You can see negative attitudes such as the hangdog 'hard-done-by' expression or the submissive or defeatist look displayed in a poor posture. Anger often gets lodged in a tight chest. There is a close relationship between poor posture and body mechanics easily observed by those around us. Sadness goes with a head dropped forward; or notice the familiar hunched shoulders of the shy or introverted personality. Posture is often associated with mood – the erect, outgoing confident stride or the self-conscious stoop. It sends out important signals to others – it can even elicit a negative response as it is clearly linked to self-esteem.

Lack of exercise is another cause of poor posture. The muscles are not worked enough and stay weak and in less-than-optimum condition. Too many of us live at this level of under-performance – we do not want to be like this, but our desire to be fit gets lost among the harsh demands of modern society. Back pain is the result of years of the quiet erosion of our true physical capacity; we remain unaware of how things really are until we feel pain as our bodies try instinctively to adapt, compromise and compensate. Stronger muscles take over to shore up weaker ones and the whole structure is placed at risk of distortion and displacement. Ageing appears to dry us out but this need not be inevitable – exercise and stretching can counteract disc shrinkage and muscle tightness that come with decreased activity. Poor posture is not inescapable and much can be done to help counter its ravages.

Types of Poor Posture

Posture classifications depend for the most part upon the spinal configuration – where and how the curves occur. Remember the spine should be a gentle S-shape without the final tail. There are several kinds of recognized posture defects (with considerable overlap and different possible combinations), based on the precise area and type of spinal curvature. For our purposes, to keep matters simple, we will confine ourselves to describing the major faults commonly seen.

Our first group of people exhibiting a common posture fault could be described as the STOOPERS or SLUMPERS. The main points to note about this group are: increased lower back curve – round shoulders often with weak abdominal muscles carrying a pot-belly; the pelvis is tilted but sagging. Breathing is often of poor quality as the chest appears sunken. The head position is usually poor; the head is often carried forward of the vertical axis, appearing to sink down between the shoulder-blades. The back curves in general are exaggerated. This combination of posture faults is common in desk workers, students – even young schoolchildren – assembly-line workers and shop-workers, and the overall impression is one of partial collapse.

This group in all its variations is by far the biggest we encounter.

Our next major group is the one that demonstrates the parade-ground, military or rigid posture – we could call the people in this group the PUSHERS or THRUSTERS. The main points about this group are that: everything is exaggerated in the opposite direction to the Slumpers. There is tightness and tension visible all over the body – the head is generally pulled way back with the chin up – the back is stiff and straight as the spine and shoulders are pulled back. The chest is thrust out and up, limiting the natural movement of the ribcage and diaphragm. This one looks better in theory, but everything is too tight and tense. The head position is often behind the vertical axis. Enormous muscular effort is required to maintain this rigidity. The spinal curves are too flat compared with the excessive curvature of the Slumpers.

These are the real extremes of poor posture, with other categories being more limited or strictly defined in their defects. Most of us have minor variations on these themes as perfect posture is rare indeed. The key to most posture faults lies in the position and movement of the head as it controls vertical pull.

Other posture faults to watch out for include:

- Head pulling back and down – very common fault, the correction of which lies at the heart of the Alexander technique.
- Shoulders hunched up and rounded forward or pulled back too far.
- Too much muscular tension visible.

We can all identify with posture defects, to a greater or lesser degree, along these lines.

Consequences of Poor Posture

Poor posture is at the root of a host of problems, from minor aches and pains to more serious conditions.

Here are a few to consider:

Low Back Pain
This is often the first effect of poor posture. The spinal curves act as shock absorbers and, if they are thrown out of their correct shape, the jarring effect can be serious. You frequently get increased muscle tension here. Disc troubles too are common and even joint collapse in the spine.

Impaired Breathing and Circulation
This is associated with a collapsed chest and upper-body concavity plus round shoulders. This restricts lung capacity and directly affects oxygen intake, leading to risk of fatigue and an all-round loss of energy. It is more difficult for a chronic Slumper to expand the chest as muscles have become tight and short and ribcage   25

elevation is restricted. Breathing quality is impaired, as carbon dioxide elimination is also reduced.

Loss of Height
This occurs, along with the slumping effect, when we are in a state of constant excessive muscular tension. Discs shrink as they dry out and we tend not to recover the lost height so readily in sleep if we have not consciously dealt with tension through exercise. We become almost fixed into tight muscle patterns.

Neck and Shoulder Pain and Headaches
These often go with the poked-forward head position. The neck and back muscles tense up to take the extra strain of holding the head in this way – very tiring over any length of time. When the head is not balanced correctly, the stress generated in the neck has to be compensated for elsewhere, and the upper-back curves are increased while the knees may lock to help take the strain. Hunched shoulders restrict head and neck movement until we find that we cannot turn our head to one side as easily as the other. As we tighten up from constant stooping, it becomes more difficult to straighten up. It is not easy to avoid this chronic head-forward position at work, and jaw problems, even migraines and associated aches and pains can be traced to this source.

Mood and Personality
Poor posture is closely associated with mood and personality as we have touched on before. How you move and hold yourself reveals and probably influences how you are feeling. Your body's signals affect the way people react towards you. This is a fascinating area of observation which is not yet treated with the importance it warrants.

Fatigue
Chronic fatigue is common and a much underrated consequence of poor posture. We take on the appearance of being worn down with responsibilities. As a result of poor-posture fatigue we may find ourselves having to work harder than necessary to perform tasks, we tighten up our 'armour' even more and carry it around

like a burden. Our body does its best to adapt to this distortion by working around it, as it were: a pattern of shortened, tight muscles emerges with corresponding long, weak muscles compensating them.

Poor posture is so noticeable that it is instantly identifiable – almost like a fingerprint. You can often recognize someone from a distance; poor posture is a difficult personal feature to disguise. As we have tried to demonstrate, it is almost impossible to function at your best when your posture is poor and, at worst, the consequences can be harmful.

However, it is comforting to know that we can almost always help ourselves by doing exercises designed specifically for posture improvement and back strengthening.

6 Stretching and Flexibility

We understand flexibility as the ability to take joints and muscles through a full range of movement – an ability which is improved by proper stretching exercises, as far as the working joint and associated muscles and ligaments will allow. We all get stiffer with age and, unless we take action, muscles tend to shorten which decreases the range of motion of the joints and we 'dry out' almost, as our tissues dehydrate and become fixed. What we are aiming for is enough flexibility to be able easily to turn, stretch, bend and twist as we wish. Until quite recently stretching has been a much undervalued part of fitness. Regular, simple stretches easily performed and fitted into the daily routine will prove to be a great help. There is no need for a break in the day's events: in fact, you are more likely to stick to the exercises when there is no need for special classes or equipment.

How to Stretch

The first step, paradoxically, is to relax, as this enables the muscles to be stretched fully. If you stretch too far or too fast, the stretch reflex is triggered and achieves the opposite effect to the one required. We need slow, static, gentle stretches – there are several in the exercise section at the back of the book.

- Warm up with a few gentle exercises (see pp. 7-9).
- Perform the stretch exercise – try to breathe out as you do this.
- Stretch only until you feel mild tension – then hold the position for between ten and thirty seconds. You will be able to hold the stretch longer as you become used to the effort. If you feel anything more than mild tension, then ease back slightly.
- Concentrate on what you are trying to achieve.
- Always stretch slowly and smoothly and do not hold your breath.

After a few weeks of practice, when you have reached the full extent of a stretch, as you relax at that point you will find that you can actually reach a little further and feel the muscles relaxing even more. The idea is to stretch to the point of very mild tension. Never force stretches, as pain comes from muscles resisting letting go and being overstretched from a cold start. By training and repetition, you will find that the critical mark where you can stretch further without pain will take longer to reach. The muscles relax and the tissues adapt. Stretching lubricates the whole system and helps it to work smoothly. To be effective, the stretches need to be held at the point of maximum resistance at the end of the normal range of movement. As we have said, this point or level is further away each time and you can actually see and feel the improvement. This is as far as you need to go and this gentle deliberate stretching, done gradually and consistently, allows slow, steady relaxation. Always use slow, static stretches as they are not only the easiest to do but also the most helpful as well as being the safest. Do not attempt vigorous or bouncing stretches such as repeated toe touches, as they activate the stretch reflex where the muscle in question contracts automatically as a protective reflex.

Benefits of Stretching

- Decreased risk of back pain and muscle soreness owing to a wider range of movement.
- Decreased risk of joint stiffness and immobility.
- Increased relaxation both mental and physical.
- Heightened sense of well-being and raised energy level as the body is toned up.
- Improved circulation.
- Enhanced personal appearance as posture improves.

Stretch just as often as you can – it is bound to vary from day to day. Stick to it, as the more you practise, the better you will get. Keep it simple and try not to get bogged down with strict timetables and exercise imperatives. It is far less hassle when you fit it in when it suits your schedule, but try to ensure that you do the stretches regularly.

We need two types of exercises to achieve the best results:

1 Stretches for flexibility and posture development.
2 Strengthening exercises to maintain new flexibility and improved posture.

7 More About Your Back – Some Useful Tips

Repetitive Strain Injury (RSI)

RSI is an umbrella definition for a wide range of disorders mainly affecting the hands, wrists, arms, neck, shoulders and back, and involving the muscles, nerves and joints. It is becoming increasingly common especially among office-workers, VDU operators, assembly-line workers and anyone whose occupation involves the constant repetition of certain actions. In view of the growing concern about health and safety standards in the workplace generally, it seems likely that official guidelines will be reinforced by legislation possibly leading to hefty penalties for those organizations that contravene them. Yet with the best will in the world, the experts can only do so much to help. Most design is a compromise aimed at the 'average' person but we all vary considerably in height, shape, size and habits: surely it makes sense for us to combat the rigours of the workplace ourselves. Defending our backs by means of a few easy exercises and stretches, incorporated without fuss into our normal routine, will go a long way towards mitigating muscular stresses and strains produced during the working day.

The more companies do to protect themselves and their employees, the better it will be for everyone concerned. Many companies are aware of this and are keen to help. Often, the solutions are simple – it can be something as elementary as the rearrangement of the working environment – listening and taking an active interest and anticipating trouble spots. There now exist comprehensive directives, introduced by the Health and Safety Executive in December 1992, regarding working conditions for VDU operators embracing everything from screens and keyboards to desks and chairs. Wider aspects of the office environment have been identified too such as lighting and humidity levels and other office equipment. There is plenty of scope for self-defence.

31

Standing Tips

- Alter your position from time to time – don't stay anchored to the same spot.
- Shift your weight about from one leg to the other and circle your feet, one foot in front of the other.
- Clasp your hands behind your back to open out your chest – *à la* royalty.
- Stroll about as much as you can without being disruptive.
- Lean back against the wall.
- Practise the Wall Stand (the PT standing).
- Rest one foot up on a chair rung (remember the saloon-bar footrail is there to make patrons feel more relaxed).
- Arch your back regularly as shown in the exercises – gently.
- Walk tall and look the world in the eyes – as the song has it.
- Keep knees slightly flexed, never locked.
- Always keep shoulders relaxed and down.
- Finally, remember the puppet on a string – lift your head straight up, chin level – elongate yourself.

Sitting Tips

- Always sit back as far as you can in the chair, especially one with a back – keep your back straight and supported.
- Use a lumbar wedge or lower-back support to eliminate the lower back hollow. Keep knees as high or higher than hips if possible.
- Use a footrest – a telephone directory will do – anything to help you to keep the pelvic tilt.
- Armrests are a good idea.

If you use an office chair, make sure it is fully adjustable and can support you in all ways – height, tilt, backrest. The seat itself should reach no more than two-thirds of the way along the length of your thighs with your feet firmly on the floor or footrest. It should provide substantial support in the lower back area. Pressure on the spine is greatest when sitting and least when lying down.

If your desk work is considerable, try an adjustable sloping work surface which is less tiring to use than a horizontal worktop. Use a stand to support the work in progress so that you can see it easily without squinting or straining. Make sure there is proper lighting.

Try to work with your forearms parallel to the table; arrange things to make life easier for yourself. Get up and move around every half-hour or so – do a few exercises from the back of the book – and break up your routine. Inject as much variety as possible into your daily tasks and try not to become tied to the desk. Stand up for telephone calls. Move about as much as you can manage. Slumping is far more tiring than sitting properly as it puts more pressure on the back and discs. As your body adapts quickly to furniture being used, it is essential to use well-designed furniture.

When sitting on a sofa, use a pillow or cushion behind your lower back to provide extra support – many easy chairs and sofas are too soft and encourage slumping.

TIP: when getting up from a seat, always straighten your back first, lead with your head and then stand up.

The greatest strain on a back in normal everyday situations comes from prolonged sitting and leaning over a desk or worktop.

Tips for Driving and Travelling

The same criteria apply to seats in cars, as for office chairs. You need a fully adjustable seat for height, back rake and fore-and-aft adjustment so that all the controls are within easy reach. Again, use a lower-back support, cushion or wedge. Many people use these special back supports. There are different types available, so experiment to find one that suits you. Stop frequently on long journeys – get out and walk around and do a few exercises. Break up the journey into easy 'bites' so that you keep tiredness at bay.

You cannot do much about the seats provided on trains, buses and aircraft but you can use the back wedges often supplied or take your own along with you. You can get up and walk about too which is equally important to keep your circulation flowing as well as to ease your back. Don't just accept what is offered without question if it does not suit you – arrange your seating to suit yourself.

Tips for Lifting, Bending and General Back Protection

- Always keep the object being lifted as close to the body as possible, using the lightest grip necessary.
- Take the strain with your thigh muscles: come down to the

loads, bending your knees to lower the centre of gravity. Do not bend at the waist as this throws enormous strain on the spine.

- Never turn and twist at the same time as lifting. If turning while load-carrying, pivot your feet in the same direction. Never turn with your load against stationary feet.
- Lower the load with the same care – or drop it.
- Never attempt to bend with locked knees – always bend your legs, never your back, so that you are not using the back muscles to do the lifting. Leg muscles are big and strong, so use them.
- Always keep the pelvic tilt and brace the abdominal muscles, although this is an instinctive action.
- Spread the load if possible – use two bags instead of one. Try to avoid carrying a shoulder-bag on one shoulder constantly: it is almost impossible to avoid tipping up the shoulder slightly to stop the bag falling off. If you must use one, put the strap on the other shoulder so that it is slung across the body.

Poor technique in these areas puts enormous unnecessary strain on the back – always think first about the easiest way to carry out any task. Use a stepladder for tasks above shoulder-height.

Lifting – Summary of Tips to Protect the Back
- Keep your back straight – squat or crouch down to pick up the load.
- Do not twist and turn when lifting.
- Grasp the load firmly – test the weight first and use the appropriate strength required. Never use fingers only.
- Keep your elbows close to your sides to stabilize the load.
- Tighten the abdominal muscles as you take the strain – keep the PT.
- Use the power of your legs to do the work – never the back – and never pick up loads away from your body. It is asking for trouble.

Back pain is common in some jobs such as nursing where it is difficult to avoid the massive leverage effect involved in lifting patients often at arm's length.

The same basic guidelines apply to housework or gardening – just work within the confines of your capacity for lifting and stretching and vary your movements. It is impossible to cater for all situations with specific instructions, so think first to avoid trouble.

Some other useful tips:

Using the Telephone
When using the telephone, resist the temptation to cradle it between your head and shoulder – it may look cool in films but is harmful over long periods.

Squatting
Learn to squat occasionally during the day. Start by holding on to the edge of a desk or worktop. Try to keep both feet flat on the floor. Use small squats at first and never go down into deep squats. Keep your back straight.

Rocking-chairs
Use one whenever you get the opportunity. It is excellent therapy for your back as it varies the load on the back muscles. It helps you to relax as well as keep the circulation going.

Deep Breathing
Stand or sit erect. Place your hands on your sides as far up towards your ribs as you can, with thumbs to the back. Breathe in, relax as you do and then gently squeeze your sides as you exhale.

Raised Desks and Writing Slopes
These are similar to a draughtsman's table and provide a suitable angled surface to work at. You can either stand at the raised surface or sit on a high stool with a footrest. They are much more comfortable than many flat-topped desks.

Relaxation
Learn some relaxation skills to ease tension – it provides valuable back-up to the exercises themselves (see Further Reading).

Beds
A great deal of information is available about beds and mattresses,

some of which is helpful. A bed can be too hard as well as too soft. The best thing to do is experiment to find out what suits you. Some exercises can be done in bed, though they are seldom as effective. The best way to get out of bed is to roll on to your side and swing your legs over the side of the bed and on to the floor. Then straighten up to a sitting position, lead with your head, keep your back straight and stand up.

Reading
Prop up a book to read – do not squint or bend your head if you can avoid it. Try an old-fashioned lectern or book-rest. If you like reading in bed, you will find it far easier if you use two pillows on your lap to rest your forearms and elbows – far less tiring. Support your back properly, of course.

Home Computers
Arrange everything to your complete satisfaction to make life easier; the correct chair, lighting, work-feed and so on.

Exercise Bar
Try to use an exercise bar where you can just hang by your arms and feel your spine stretch. Anything to get your feet off the ground, which rehydrates the spinal discs; you even feel taller immediately.

Posture Chairs or Kneeling Chairs
These may be useful – some people swear by them, while others cannot get on with them at all.

Emergency Treatment for an Attack of Back Pain
1 Stop what you are doing and, if possible, rest.
2 Apply an ice-pack to the affected area and keep this on for ten to twenty minutes. Repeat every two to three hours. (Use a packet of vegetables from the freezer but wrap it in a towel first to prevent cold burns.)
3 Take bedrest if possible, but no longer than is strictly necessary – as soon as you are able, get up and move around.
4 Start gentle exercises and resolve to pursue a preventive programme to reduce the risk of further attacks.

8 In Conclusion

The old saying 'A penny of prevention is worth a pound of cure', is as true for back pain as it is for anything else. The best preventive measure for your back is a regular exercise programme to stretch and strengthen your back and abdominal muscles. In addition, acquire good posture habits to reinforce back protection. Back pain is usually the long-term result of poor posture combined with a lack of general physical fitness. Remember that ninety per cent of back pain is non-specific and can be dealt with fairly easily if consideration is given to posture and exercise. You can take the initiative and not remain a passive victim. It really is up to you to protect your own back. Learn the basic guidelines and care for your back on a daily basis.

Steps to Take

- Think POSTURE until it has become a relaxed habit – check it frequently throughout the day. Keep the pelvic tilt or do the Wall Stand whenever possible.
- Strengthen your abdominal and back muscles to render you less vulnerable to injury.
- Exercise your joints – take them regularly through their full range of movement – every day if possible.
- Develop an awareness of your back in your daily routine, and resolve to protect it.

The Exercises

Arm Circles

PURPOSE

Loosens up shoulder girdle and opens up chest area.
Use also as a warm-up exercise.

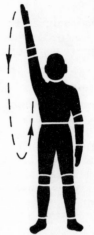

METHOD

1 Stand tall with a good posture and pelvic tilt with
  your arms at your sides.
2 Keep your feet a shoulder-width apart.
3 Move both arms backward in slow full circles,
  making as wide a circle as possible while you feel
  the stretch all round.
4 Circle backward first, then forward.
5 Use one arm at a time to begin with then circle
  both arms like a propeller in different directions,
  starting with one arm up and one arm down.
6 Keep hands open and breathe easily and normally.
7 Describe as large a circle as possible.

Arm Circles Variation

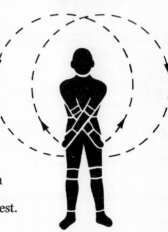

METHOD

1 Stand tall with a good posture and pelvic tilt.
2 Let both arms dangle loosely at your sides.
3 Inhale deeply and cross both arms in front
  of your body, feeling the stretch in your
  shoulder-blades.
4 Lift your crossed arms up over your head.
5 Exhale slowly and bring your arms round in an
  arc behind your body.
6 Lower them and feel the stretch across your chest.
7 Repeat ten times.
8 Vary this by using one arm at a time.

POINTS TO NOTE

1 Keep spine long, stand tall and keep a good pelvic tilt.
2 Keep arms close to ears and describe wide, slow circles.
3 *Do not shake or move* your body and breathe normally.

41

Ceiling Reaches

PURPOSE

To loosen up arms and shoulder muscles.
To stretch sides and chest and relieve tension.
A superb warm-up exercise.

METHOD

1 Stand with your feet a shoulder-width apart.
2 Keep a good posture and pelvic tilt.
3 With your left hand on your hip, extend your right
   arm overhead and reach up as far as you can
   towards the ceiling.
4 Alternate arms ten times each.
5 Use your arms singly to begin with then use both
   arms together.
6 Try to stretch higher and higher and feel your
   spine lengthen.

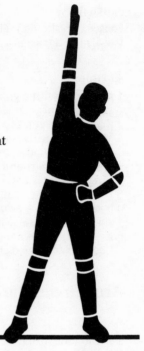

Ceiling Reaches Variation

METHOD

1 Stand tall with a good posture and pelvic tilt.
2 Place feet a shoulder-width apart.
3 Interlock your hands overhead.
4 Stretch up with your palms facing the ceiling.
5 Try to stretch as high as you can, *but do not
   overstretch.*

POINTS TO NOTE

1 Do not arch your back.
2 Keep your shoulders loose and down.
3 Either hold each stretch at the top or alternate in steady rhythm
   for warming up.
4 Keep your head facing forward or look up at the ceiling.

Side Bends

PURPOSE

To stretch sides and waist and key postural muscles.
To mobilize spine and trim waistline.

METHOD

1 Stand with feet a shoulder-width apart and knees
   slightly flexed.
2 Keep a good pelvic tilt.
3 Raise your right arm over your head and place
   your left arm across in front of your abdomen.
4 Stretch slowly over to the left as far as you can
   easily go while extending your right arm over to a
   diagonal position.
5 Hold for a slow count of ten as you feel the stretch
   down your side.
6 Repeat twice then change sides and arms and
   repeat twice on that side.

Side Bends Variation

METHOD

1 Instead of placing one arm across your abdomen,
   place it on one hip to help the bend as you push
   into your hip.
2 As you get stronger, you will be able to bend further.

POINTS TO NOTE

1 Keep shoulders in one plane with hips; arms and head in one plane
   with shoulders – do not bend forward.
2 Breathe out as you do the stretch.
3 Try to keep your raised arm close to your ear.
4 *Do not arch your back.*
5 Stop the exercise if you feel resistance and gradually increase the
   stretch only when it feels comfortable.
6 Do the exercise slowly and gently.

43

Hip Circles

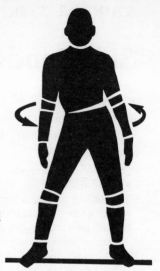

PURPOSE

To loosen up your lower back.

METHOD

1 Stand tall with a good posture and pelvic tilt.
2 Place your feet a shoulder-width apart.
3 Let arms hang free or place on hips.
4 Circle hips, first to one side then to the back and then to the other side and then to the front and then again to the side to complete the circle.
5 Repeat exercise five times in each direction.

Hip Circles Variation

METHOD

1 Stand tall with a good posture and pelvic tilt.
2 Place feet a shoulder-width apart.
3 Place both hands on hips.
4 Swing hips first to one side then the other in pendulum fashion.
5 Hold at each side for a count of ten, then swing to the other side.
6 Repeat exercise five times.

POINTS TO NOTE

1 Always keep knees loosely flexed.
2 Roll pelvis round in as big a circle as possible.
3 Try to use your abdominal muscles to help you.
4 Keep your shoulders still and relaxed.

Half Knee Bends

PURPOSE

Good for calves, thigh muscles and posture.

METHOD

1 Stand with a good posture.
2 Place hands on hips.
3 Take a half-step forward with one foot and a half-step back with the other foot so that your feet are about twelve inches apart, toes facing forward.
4 Bend the front knee.
5 Keep your back leg straight and both feet flat on the floor.
6 Hold for a count of ten and feel the stretch in the calf muscle of the back leg.
7 Repeat the exercise, starting with your other foot forward.

Half Knee Bends Variation

METHOD

1 Stand up straight with your feet together.
2 Stretch your arms out in front of you at shoulder-level.
3 Bend your knees, keeping your feet flat on the floor.
4 Return to starting position, relax and repeat.
5 Repeat this exercise until you feel your thigh muscles aching slightly. Hold as long as you can easily.
6 *Do not bend your knees too far. Never go down any further than forty-five degrees.*
7 This exercise tightens your quadricep muscles and relaxes the hamstrings.

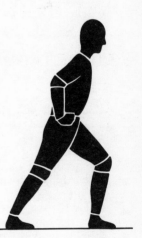

POINTS TO NOTE

1 Breathe out as you bend your knees in both exercises.
2 Keep body upright throughout.
3 *Do not bend too far.*

45

Trunk Twists

PURPOSE

To mobilize spine and waist and generally loosen up.

METHOD

1 Stand tall with your feet a shoulder-width apart.
2 Keep a good posture and pelvic tilt with your knees flexed.
3 Slowly twist your trunk first round to the left then round to the right as far as you can go with ease.
4 Hold that position for a count of ten.
5 Repeat, twisting first to the right then to the left.
6 Relax, then repeat the exercise five times.

Trunk Twists Variation

METHOD

1 Stand tall with your feet a shoulder-width apart.
2 Keep a good posture and pelvic tilt with your knees flexed.
3 You can vary the exercise either by placing your fingertips on your shoulders, your hands on your hips or linking your outstretched hands in front of you.
4 Slowly twist your trunk first to the left, then to the right as far as you can go with ease.
5 Hold that position for a count of ten.
6 Repeat, twisting first to the right then to the left.
7 Relax, then repeat the exercise.

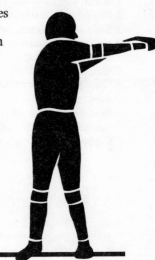

POINTS TO NOTE

1 Keep hips and knees steady.
2 Move slowly and gently.
3 Keep a good pelvic tilt.
4 *Do not lock your knees.*

Slumps

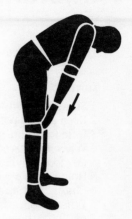

PURPOSE

Good exercise for relaxation and loosening up.

METHOD

1 Stand tall with a good posture, feet slightly apart.
2 Bend your head and put your chin on your chest.
3 Slide hands down your legs towards your knees.
4 Curl yourself down to follow hands as far as you can easily go. This is *not* toe touching.
5 Relax neck and shoulders.
6 Let your neck muscles go loose.
7 Return to an upright position by uncoiling upward.

Slumps Variation

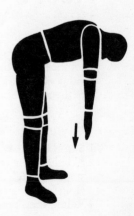

METHOD

1 Stand tall with a good posture, feet apart, knees slightly flexed.
2 Start with your hands overhead and let your arms hang loose as you curl down.
3 Bend forward. *Do not try to touch the floor.*
4 Hang in that position totally relaxed, heavy and loose.
5 Hold for a slow count of ten.
6 Using your thigh muscles to propel yourself, return to an upright position.
7 As you come up, stretch your hands and arms overhead towards the ceiling.
8 Breathe out as you go down and inhale as you come up.

POINTS TO NOTE

1 Let head come down and over towards the floor, allowing your body to curl down.
2 Keep your chin tucked in to lengthen your neck.

47

Standing on Tiptoe

PURPOSE

To strengthen calves and improve balance.

METHOD

1 Stand normally and rise up on tiptoe.
2 Keep a good posture with pelvic tilt.
3 Hold for a slow count of ten then repeat.
4 When this exercise becomes too easy, rise up on one foot only, keeping the other foot off the ground.
5 Hold for a slow count of ten.
6 Change feet and repeat.
7 When this too becomes easy, try to walk around on tiptoe, holding on to a support if necessary.

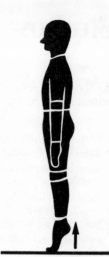

Heel Drops

PURPOSE

Strengthens the calves and improves the balance. Stretches heel tendons which are essential for good posture. You can do these Heel Drops after practising the Standing on Tiptoe exercise.

METHOD

1 Stand on the edge of a step.
2 Slowly lower your heels over the edge of the step to stretch.
3 Hold for fifteen to twenty seconds.
4 Relax, then repeat exercise.

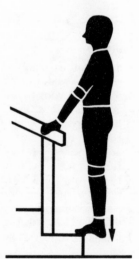

POINTS TO NOTE

1 Keep feet slightly apart to aid balance.
2 Rise up as high as you can go, *but do not strain.*
3 Lower heels very slowly.

48

Arching Back

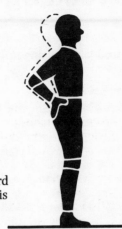

PURPOSE

Relieves backache and tension, especially for
sedentary workers.

METHOD

1 Stand with a good posture and your feet a
  shoulder-width apart.
2 Place your hands in the small of your back.
3 Breathe in deeply.
4 Breathe out slowly while gently bending backward
  and supporting your back with your hands. This is
  gentle back arching. *Do not arch your back too far.*
5 Repeat five times.

> **POINTS TO NOTE**
>
> 1 *Do not arch your back too far* as this compresses the spinal joints,
>   which can be very bad for your back.
> 2 Take things easily at all times.

Leg Swings on Box

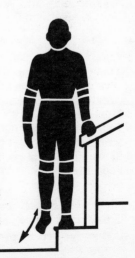

PURPOSE

Loosens up hips and helps leg circulation.

METHOD

1 Stand on a low box or bottom stair.
2 Swing one leg freely back and forth.
3 Let the leg relax and use its own weight to exert
  mild traction.
4 Describe small arcs at first and gradually extend
  the arc as you do the exercise.
5 Change legs and repeat the exercise.

49

Wood Chopper

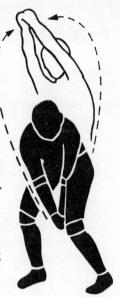

PURPOSE

Good for loosening up and warming up.

METHOD

1 Stand tall with your feet apart.
2 Clasp both hands together over your head.
3 Swing your arms down through your legs, bending at the knees and waist as if you were chopping wood.
4 Repeat ten times.
5 As a variation, keep hands a shoulder-width apart and do the exercise swinging your arms down and outside your legs instead of between them.
6 Continue by straightening your knees and swinging your arms forward and up to reach for the ceiling.
7 Do not rush this exercise and take it gently.

Chest Arm Flings

PURPOSE

Loosening up shoulders and arms and warming up.

METHOD

1 Stand with your feet a shoulder-width apart.
2 Keep your elbows out at shoulder-level with your arms in so that fingers touch in front of your chest.
3 Press shoulders back so fingers no longer touch.
4 Touch fingers together again then throw your arms out and back at the same height.
5 Return to the first position.
6 Repeat ten times.

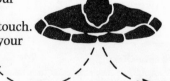

POINTS TO NOTE

Do these exercises slowly and properly. Remember, you are *not in a race*.

Hamstring Stretch

PURPOSE

To stretch hamstrings, which is essential for good posture, walking, standing and lifting.
To develop leg strength.

METHOD

1 Use a low stool for this exercise. *Do not use a table as it will be much too high and can adversely affect your back.*
2 Face stool and place your left heel on it, standing straight with the knee flexed.
3 Bend forward very gently. Experiment with this position to feel the stretch (you will probably feel it immediately).
4 Hold on to a tabletop if you wish to aid your balance.
5 When you feel comfortable, you can increase the stretch by pushing down hard with the heel of your outstretched leg as if you are trying to push the stool into the floor.
6 Hold for a slow count of ten.
7 Relax and very gently let your heel slide farther away from you until it feels tight again. You may have to bend the supporting knee more as you lean forward gently.
8 Change legs and repeat.

POINTS TO NOTE

1 *Do not lock either knee.*
2 Keep the pelvic tilt with your head and trunk long.
3 Keep outstretched foot on a *low* stool or similar chair. If the surface is too high you will overstretch your lower back and pull your pelvis out of line.
4 Use a wall or similar to support yourself.

51

Arms Out Front

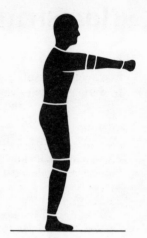

PURPOSE

To stretch upper back and generally loosen up.

METHOD

1 Stand tall with a good posture and knees flexed.
2 Keep a good pelvic tilt.
3 Interlock your fingers and push your hands out from your chest at shoulder-level.
4 Round upper back slightly and look down at the floor.
5 Hold for a slow count of ten.
6 Release and repeat the exercise.

Foot Up

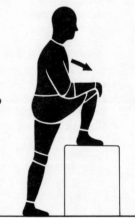

PURPOSE

To ease lower back and hip tension.

METHOD

1 Select table, worktop or desk, etc., but nothing too high. You will have to experiment for yourself.
2 Place one foot up on the surface, keeping your other foot flat on the floor.
3 Clasp the uplifted knee.
4 Slowly move your chest in towards your clasped knee.
5 Hold for a slow count of ten.
6 Change legs and repeat.

POINTS TO NOTE

1 *Stand tall with a good posture and pelvic tilt.*
2 **Take things easily at all times.**

Side Bends to Wall

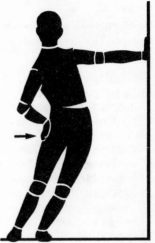

PURPOSE

To stretch your side and abdominal muscles.
To stretch and ease your spine.

METHOD

1 Stand sideways to the wall. Lift your left arm and place your palm on the wall at about shoulder-level.
2 Lean into the wall keeping outstretched arm straight.
3 Use right hand on right hip and push hip in towards the wall to help stretch torso into a bow shape. Keep feet still.
4 Hold stretch for a slow count of ten, then release. Repeat five times.
5 Change arms and stretch the other side.

Side Bends to Wall Variation

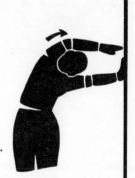

METHOD

1 Stand sideways to the wall. Lift your left arm and place your palm on the wall at about shoulder-level.
2 Stretch your right arm over your head and attempt to touch the wall without twisting or leaning.
3 Hold stretch for a slow count of ten, then release. Repeat five times.
4 Change sides and repeat.

POINTS TO NOTE

1 Keep feet slightly apart to aid balance. Keep trunk and hips still.
2 Keep knees slightly flexed *not* rigid. *Do not force.* Take things gently *at all times.*
3 Breathe normally. Inhale as you stretch and exhale as you release the stretch.

53

Wall Squats

PURPOSE

Strengthens legs and stretches Achilles tendons –
essential for good posture.

METHOD

1 Stand with your back against a smooth wall or
 door with your feet six inches away.
2 Flatten your lower back against the wall, keeping
 pelvis tilted.
3 Slide down the wall slowly until your legs are bent
 to about forty-five degrees.
4 Return to starting position.
5 Repeat until you feel mild tiredness in your legs.
6 Do not go past forty-five degrees at first until you
 find squat too easy, then gradually and easily
 deepen the squat until you can reach the position
 where your thighs are almost, but not quite,
 parallel to the floor. You need go no further with
 the squat as this just overtaxes your knee-joints.
7 Keep shoulders relaxed and down.

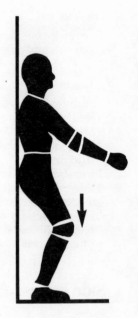

POINTS TO NOTE

1 Keep shoulders level and relaxed with the chin in and head up and
 back.
2 Keep knees flexed at the start with feet flat on the floor.
3 Do not try to bend knees farther than forty-five degrees to begin
 with as this exercise is really a wall slide.
4 Vary the distance of your feet from the wall to adjust the severity
 of the stretch and use a chair back for support at first to help
 balance and recovery.
5 This exercise is designed to strengthen the quadriceps which are
 essential for walking, standing and lifting and help posture
 immensely.

EXERCISES USING WALL OR DOOR

Wall Squats Variation 1

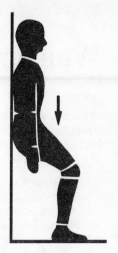

METHOD

1 This is a variation on the first Wall Squat exercise. Try both and see which one you prefer.
2 Stand with your back to the wall as before with your feet about a foot away from its surface.
3 Bend your knees and go down as if practising sitting without a chair until your back comes to rest against the wall.
4 Hold for a count of ten and then repeat.

Wall Squats Variation 2

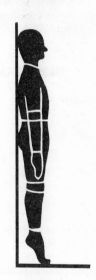

METHOD

1 Stand with heels close to the wall.
2 Flatten lower back against the wall while adopting a good position.
3 Rise up the wall until you stand on tiptoe.
4 Keep this position as your feet return flat on to the floor. (For postural improvement, try to think of an imaginary wall behind you as you walk about.)
5 When you have managed to achieve this good posture, and you will know immediately when you have it, walk away from the wall then return to the wall and see if you have kept the new position. Practise this exercise as often as you can through the day as it is a real boost to good posture.

POINTS TO NOTE

1 Keep shoulders level and relaxed with chin in and head up and back.
2 Keep pelvic tilt with tummy and buttocks in.
3 These are marvellous exercises for reducing excessive spinal curvature.

Wall Stand

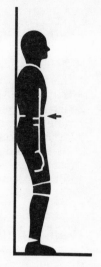

PURPOSE

Superb posture improver.
Great for strength and all-round benefit.
Helps ease neck pains and strains.

METHOD

1 Stand with your back to a wall or door with feet
   about six inches away from wall.
2 Flex knees and push your lower back against the
   wall until it touches the surface.
3 Keeping your chin level, pull your head back as
   far as you can.
4 Hold for a slow count of ten.

Wall Stand Variation 1

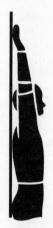

PURPOSE

Helps to correct rounded shoulders and strengthens
the back.

METHOD

1 Stand with your back to a wall as before.
2 Flatten lower back against wall as before.
3 Raise arms overhead with palms facing outwards,
   keeping the back of your hands against the wall.
4 Breathe in as you lift your arms overhead. Exhale
   as you lower arms.
5 Try to keep your hands against the wall. This is
   not easy, but persevere as you will quickly feel the
   benefit.

POINTS TO NOTE

1 Keep shoulders relaxed and down and breathe easily at all times.
2 If your head does not touch the wall at first, it soon will as you get
   stronger and your posture improves.

Wall Stand Variation 2

METHOD

1 Stand with your back to a wall with feet about six inches away from wall. If you find this too difficult, position your feet twelve inches away from the wall.
2 Flatten your lower back against the wall as before.
3 Raise your arms overhead with palms facing outwards, keeping the backs of your hands against the wall.
4 Breathe in as you lift your arms overhead. Exhale as you lower your arms.
5 Try to keep hands against the wall. This is not easy, but persevere as you will quickly feel the benefit.
6 Once you have your hands up overhead, slide them down the wall into the 'surrender' position.
7 Hold and then stretch them up again. Hold for a count of five at first.
8 Increase hold once you can actually do it. This is not easy, but do persevere as this is an enormous help to posture.
9 If you wish, you can try this exercise with your palms facing the other way.

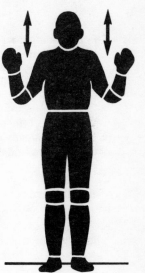

POINTS TO NOTE
Keep pelvic tilt and breathe easily at all times.

Tendon Stretches

PURPOSE

To stretch calves and Achilles tendons to help posture.

METHOD

1 Stand facing a wall about an arm's-length away.
2 Put both hands on the wall at shoulder-height.
3 Bring one leg forward, bending the knee.
4 Keep your other leg straight with the foot flat on the floor.
5 Lean forward into the wall, bending your elbows. You will feel the calf stretch in your straight leg.
6 Hold for a steady count of ten. Relax and repeat.
7 Change legs and repeat exercise.

To continue the stretch and bring it down from the calf to the tendon:

1 Adopt the same position as before.
2 This time, slightly bend the knee of the extended leg, keeping that foot firmly planted on the floor.

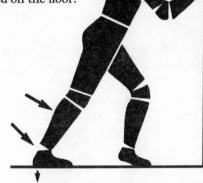

POINTS TO NOTE

1 Do this exercise gently.
2 Keep foot of extended leg flat and pointing straight towards the wall.
3 *Do not arch your back or overstretch.*
4 To vary the stretch, vary the distance from the wall with your feet.

Chest Stretches I

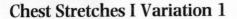

PURPOSE

To stretch chest and shoulder muscles.
To release tension in upper back and shoulders.

METHOD

1 Stand about an arm's-length away from an open doorway.
2 Place hands on door-frame at about shoulder-level.
3 Lean forward, keeping chin in and head up.
4 Feel your chest being stretched as you lean in.
5 Hold stretch for a slow count of ten then return to an upright position.
6 Move your hands up and down the door-frame and to the lintel to vary the stretch.
7 After each stretch, return to the upright position and repeat each position twice more.

Chest Stretches I Variation 1

METHOD

1 Stand almost in the doorway.
2 Place forearms on the door-frame with hands at about head-level.
3 Take a small step forward.
4 Hold for a slow count of ten then repeat.
5 Adjust the size of step to vary stretch.
6 Another variation is to walk through the door whilst keeping your hands on the door-frame.

POINTS TO NOTE

1 *Do not let your back sag inward or arch outward.*
2 Keep feet slightly apart with heels on the floor and adjust the position of the feet in order to obtain a good stretch.
3 Always keep your head up and your chin in.
4 To vary the stretch and the effect of these exercises, vary the position of your hands and feet, but always take things easy.

59

Chest Stretches I Variation 2

METHOD
1 Stand facing the corner of a room where you can get right into the corner easily with your feet.
2 Place your hands up against the two walls and allow your body to lean forward.
3 Press forward gently and feel your chest muscles working.
4 Hold for a slow count of ten.
5 Relax, then repeat the exercise.

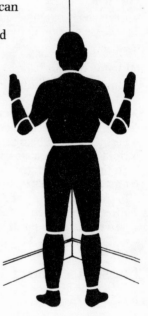

POINTS TO NOTE
See POINTS TO NOTE on p. 59

Knee to Chest I

PURPOSE

To ease backache and reduce strain and tension.

METHOD

1 Stand with your back to a wall or door.
2 Lift one knee and hug it to your chest. This
   helps to keep the lower back against the wall.
3 Hold for a count of ten.
4 Repeat the exercise with the other knee.

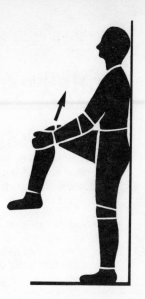

Finger Wall Walk

PURPOSE

To loosen up shoulders and open up chest.

METHOD

1 Stand facing the wall about an arm's-length
   away.
2 Starting at waist-level, walk your fingers up
   the wall as far as you can go.
3 Repeat with the other hand.
4 To vary this exercise, stand sideways to the
   wall and repeat as above.
5 Change arms and repeat.

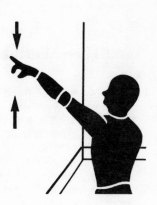

POINTS TO NOTE

1 Stand upright with your chin in and level and your head up.
2 *Do not bend or arch your back to reach further up the wall.*

Wall Turns

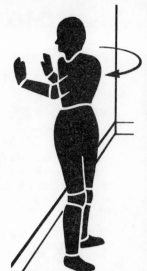

PURPOSE

To loosen up shoulder joints, back and spinal muscles and to stretch the upper body.

METHOD

1 Stand with your back to the wall with your feet a shoulder-width apart and about twelve to eighteen inches away from the wall. Keep your knees flexed.
2 Keep your hands apart and slowly turn around, placing your hands on the wall at shoulder-level.
3 Hold for a slow count of ten.
4 Return to the starting position and repeat on the other side.
5 To vary this, turn your head away from the wall once your hands are in place on the wall surface.

Wall Turns Variation

METHOD

1 Stand sideways to the wall with your feet close to the surface.
2 Place your left arm out behind you along the wall at shoulder-level with your fingers pointing away from your body.
3 Slightly turn your body out away from the wall, leaving your hand where it is. Feel the stretch along your arm and shoulder as your chest opens.
4 Hold the position for a slow count of ten.
5 Change arms and repeat the exercise.
6 Vary the stretch by turning your head away from the wall to look over your outside shoulder.
7 At the start, you may almost have to face the wall before you can turn outward, until the shoulder becomes more supple.

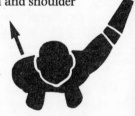

POINTS TO NOTE

1 Keep thighs, hips, knees and feet facing forward.
2 *Do not force anything. Take things slowly and gently.*

Calf Stretch

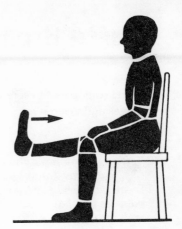

PURPOSE

Stretches legs and calf muscles.

METHOD

1 Sit up straight in a chair with a good
   pelvic tilt.
2 Extend your right leg out in front of you.
3 Try to pull your toes back towards your
   body to stretch your calf muscles.
4 Repeat the exercise with your left leg.

Ankle Circles

PURPOSE

Helps leg circulation especially in desk-bound
workers.

METHOD

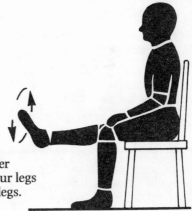

1 Sit upright in a chair and point your
   right leg straight out, keeping the
   leg straight.
2 Point your toes away from you and
   draw circles with your toes.
3 Repeat five times.
4 Relax, then repeat the exercise with
   your left leg.
5 To vary this exercise, place a waste-paper
   basket between your ankles, keeping your legs
   straight out, then raise and lower both legs.
   Relax, then repeat.

POINTS TO NOTE
Keep a good posture with a good pelvic tilt.

Seated Breathing

PURPOSE

Pure relaxation and to soothe away tension.

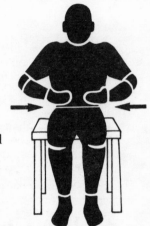

METHOD

1 Sit up straight in a chair.
2 Rest your open hands on your waist under the ribs, with your thumbs pointing to the rear.
3 Breathe in deeply and out completely, using hand pressure to help you squeeze the air out as you breathe.
4 *For a few seconds only*, keep pressure on hands as you try to inhale.
5 Release hand pressure and breathe deeply.

Body Hugs

PURPOSE

To stretch upper back and chest.

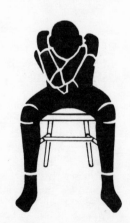

METHOD

1 Sit up in a chair with a good posture.
2 Place your hands around opposite shoulders as if hugging yourself because you are cold.
3 Bend forward towards your knees and let gravity take you down.
4 Straighten up slightly.
5 Hold the position for a count of twenty.
6 To vary this exercise, repeat the above, but turn slightly to each side.
7 Repeat the exercise.

POINTS TO NOTE

1 Do these exercises gently, breathing easily at all times.
2 Excellent exercises for relaxation and releasing tension.

Chest Stretches II

PURPOSE

Counteracts round shoulders.
Increases chest mobility and loosens shoulders.
Helps posture and opens up chest.

METHOD

1 Sit up in a chair with your back long and a good
   pelvic tilt.
2 Clasp your hands behind you at buttock-level with
   the palm of one hand lying loosely within the palm
   of the other and both palms facing the ceiling.
3 Bend your elbows slightly and keep your
   shoulders down.
4 Breathe in deeply.
5 Breathe out and squeeze your shoulder-
   blades together.
6 Close your elbows towards each other and
   feel the stretch across the chest and upper back.
7 *Do not arch your lower back too far.*
8 Repeat exercise five times.

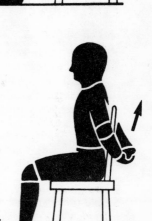

Chest Stretches II Variation

METHOD

1 Sitting on a normal office or desk chair, clasp your
   hands behind your back *and* the chair.
2 Keeping your hands clasped, raise your arms and
   hands as high as you can.
3 *Do not force your arms.*
4 Breathe in and then raise your arms a little farther.
5 Hold for a slow count of five.
6 Relax and repeat the exercise.

POINTS TO NOTE
Excellent exercises for relaxation and releasing tension.

Chest Arm Pull

PURPOSE

Eases shoulder strain.
Loosens up joints and eases upper back.

METHOD

1 Sit upright in a chair.
2 Take your right arm across your chest to grasp
  your left shoulder.
3 Grasp your right elbow with your left hand.
4 Gently pull the elbow across in front of your chest
  and let your right hand go over the back of your
  left shoulder.
5 Change arms and repeat the exercise.

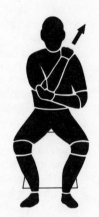

Chest Arm Pull Variation

METHOD

1 When you have got used to the previous stretch,
  vary the exercise by pulling the right elbow back
  against the pressure of your hand.
2 Adjust these positions to vary the stretch.
3 Change arms and repeat.

POINTS TO NOTE

1 *Do not overstretch yourself.*
2 Superb relaxation exercises – you will feel the benefit at once.

Chair Slumps

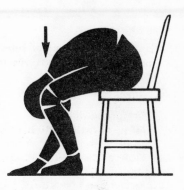

PURPOSE

Relieves aches and pains and eases tension.
Stretches lower back and helps circulation.

METHOD

1 Sit up straight on a chair.
2 Keep your feet and knees apart.
3 Bend forward towards the floor as far as
   you can go easily. Do not push down.
4 Hold for a slow count of ten.
5 Return to the starting position and repeat.
6 This is easier to do if you sit forward on the edge of
   the chair so that part of your weight is on your
   feet and legs, not all on the chair seat. Let your
   body bend and leave your arms dangling and loose.
   Let your neck and head hang too with your
   shoulders relaxed.

Chair Slumps Variation

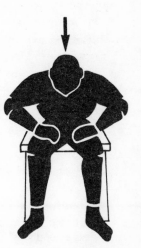

METHOD

1 Rest your palms on your thighs with fingers facing
   inward.
2 Support the weight of your upper body with your
   hands and allow your elbows to bend as your head
   and chest curve downward.
3 Hold, then gradually push your body upright.
4 Repeat five times.
5 Eventually try to get your head down near your
   knees.

POINTS TO NOTE

1 *Do not force, just hang loose.*
2 Use hands on thighs to help recovery to an upright position.
3 Allow your back to round gently.
4 Breathe easily and deeply.

67

Pelvic Slides

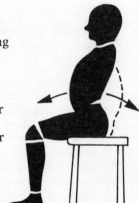

PURPOSE

To loosen up pelvis and hips.
A marvellous exercise for loosening up and relieving tension generally.

METHOD

1 Sit up straight, with a good posture, on a chair or stool.
2 Slowly and gently, arch your back and bend your spine and lower back by rocking your pelvis forward and backward.
3 Repeat at least twenty times.
4 As this exercise is easy to do anywhere, repeat as often as you can throughout the day.

POINTS TO NOTE

Do not move your position on seat.

Chair Lifts

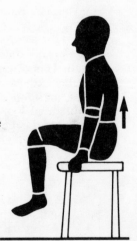

PURPOSE

To loosen up shoulders and arms.

METHOD

1 Sit in a chair or on a stool, keeping a good posture and a good pelvic tilt.
2 Place your hands on either side of the seat and grasp tightly.
3 Try to lift your body weight just off the seat by using your abdominal muscles.
4 Keep your shoulders down, arms straight.
5 *Do not tense your neck.*
6 Try to lift your feet up to clear the ground, breathing in as you do so.

Neck Turns

PURPOSE

To strengthen neck muscles.

METHOD

1 Sit up on an ordinary desk or office chair.
2 Anchor your left hand beside you under the chair seat to help keep your left shoulder down.
3 Tuck your chin in to lengthen your neck and lower your head sideways on to your right shoulder.
4 Aim your right ear at your right shoulder and feel the stretch along the left side of your neck.
5 Repeat with the other side.
6 To vary this exercise, repeat as above, but placing your right hand over your left ear before lowering your head to the right.
7 Repeat exercise from your right side.

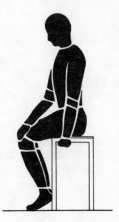

Neck Turns Variation

METHOD

1 Sit upright on an ordinary chair.
2 Anchor your left hand beside you under the chair seat to help keep your left shoulder down.
3 Turn your head about forty-five degrees to the right. Drop your chin and head down as if you were looking at the floor.
4 Hold for a count of ten and then repeat.
5 You can also put your right hand over your left ear as in the previous exercise. Repeat the whole exercise, half turning to the left.

POINTS TO NOTE
Stretch easily and gently and *do not force.*

Laced Finger Stretch

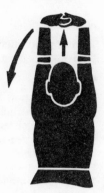

PURPOSE

To ease away upper-body tensions and backache.
To loosen up shoulders.

METHOD

1 Interlace your fingers and straighten out your
   arms in front of you at shoulder-level.
2 Keep your palms facing away from you.
3 Hold for a count of fifteen while you feel the
   stretch in your arms and shoulders.
4 To vary this exercise, stretch arms upward instead
   of straight out so that your palms face the ceiling.
   Keep your fingers interlaced and feel the stretch
   upward.

Finger Stretch Variation

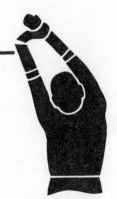

METHOD

1 Keep arms overhead, but release finger interlock.
2 This time, grasp left hand with right hand and
   pull your left arm over your head to the right side.
3 Keep both arms straight.
4 Feel your ribcage and chest open out and up and
   your spine lengthen.
5 Hold for a slow count of ten, then relax.
6 Change arms, then repeat.
7 Repeat the exercise as you feel the benefit.

POINTS TO NOTE

1 *Do not overstretch yourself.*
2 Excellent exercise for releasing tension.

Shoulder Circles

PURPOSE

Mobilizes shoulders and loosens upper-back muscles.
Relieves upper-back tension.

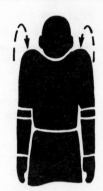

METHOD

1 Stand with a good posture and feet slightly apart.
2 Circle both shoulders by rounding them forward,
  lifting them up towards the ceiling then pulling
  them back.
3 Relax: let them fall back to the starting position.
4 Repeat in the opposite direction.
5 Repeat the exercise ten times, alternating shoulders.

Shoulder Circles Variation

METHOD

1 Stand with a good posture and feet slightly apart.
2 Keeping your arms relaxed, raise your right
  shoulder towards your right ear and circle your
  shoulder backward and forward and up and down.
3 Repeat with the left shoulder.
4 Use one shoulder first then the other, then circle in
  the opposite direction.
5 Repeat the exercise using both shoulders together.
6 To vary this, bring your left shoulder up towards
  your left ear and drop it down again.
7 Move your shoulders up and down smoothly.
8 Repeat using your right shoulder, then using both
  shoulders together.

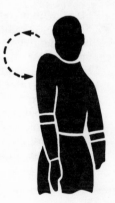

POINTS TO NOTE

1 *Do not tense shoulders as you move them.*
2 Keep your arms relaxed and hanging loose.
3 Make circles slow and well-controlled and as big as possible.
4 Keep knees flexed, with your head up and your chin in.
5 Keep your chest still and your spine straight.

71

Shoulder Shrugs

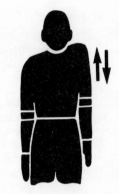

PURPOSE

Mobilizes shoulders and loosens upper-back muscles.
Relieves upper-back tension.

METHOD

1 Stand with a good posture and feet slightly apart.
2 Shrug your right shoulder up towards your right ear.
3 Repeat with your left shoulder.
4 Relax, then repeat using both shoulders together.
5 Repeat the exercise ten times.

Shoulder Shrugs Variation

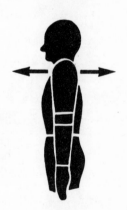

METHOD

1 Stand with a good posture and feet slightly apart.
2 Shrug your right shoulder up towards your right ear and move your shoulder backward and forward.
3 Relax and repeat with your left shoulder.
4 When you relax each shrug, consciously let your shoulders relax further than normal as if they were sinking down.
5 Using both shoulders together, repeat the exercise.
6 Repeat ten times.
7 Combine all these exercises and feel the tension disappear.

POINTS TO NOTE

1 *Do not tense shoulders as you move them.*
2 Keep your arms relaxed and hanging loose.
3 Do the exercises smoothly and slowly.
4 Keep knees flexed, with your head up and your chin in.
5 Keep your chest still and your spine straight.

Hands Behind Back

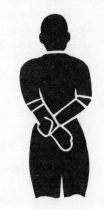

PURPOSE

To stretch shoulders and upper back.
To ease away tension.

METHOD

1 Stand or sit.
2 Put both arms out behind you.
3 Grasp one wrist with the other hand.
4 Pull both arms out away from you as far as you
  comfortably can.
5 Hold for a slow count of ten.
6 Change arms and repeat.
7 Repeat exercise five times.

Hands Behind Back Variation 1

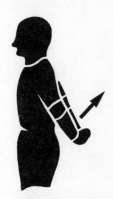

METHOD

1 Stand or sit with both arms straight out behind you.
2 Instead of clasping one wrist with the other hand,
  interlock your fingers behind your back.
3 Keeping your arms straight, inhale as you lift your
  arms out away from your body.
4 Lift your arms as high as you can with ease and
  squeeze your shoulder-blades together.
5 Hold outstretched position for a count of ten.
6 Exhale as you lower your arms, letting your
  elbows bend.
7 Repeat exercise five times.

POINTS TO NOTE

1 Stand or sit well with a good pelvic tilt. *Do not arch your back.*
2 *Do not slump forward*; this will reduce the effectiveness of the stretch.
3 Keep arms straight and lift them as high as you can with ease.
4 Feel the stretch across your arms, shoulders and chest muscles.
5 Keep your knees slightly flexed.

Hands Behind Back Variation 2

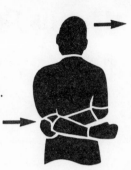

METHOD

1 Stand or sit and put your arms straight out behind you.
2 Take hold of your elbow or forearm with one hand.
3 Gently pull your arm downward so that your shoulder is depressed.
4 At the same time, tilt your head to the opposite side from the arm which you are pulling until you feel a mild stretch down your neck and shoulder.
5 Hold for a count of ten, relax, then change arms.
6 Repeat the exercise five times.

POINTS TO NOTE

1 Stand or sit well with a good pelvic tilt. *Do not arch your back.*
2 Feel the stretch across your arms, shoulders and chest muscles.
3 Keep your knees slightly flexed.

Tabletop Dips

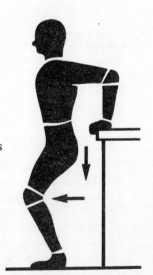

PURPOSE

Strengthens and loosens up shoulder and chest muscles and eases upper back.

METHOD

1 Stand with your back to a solid work surface.
2 Place your hands on the surface.
3 Bend your knees and drop down to the floor as far as your shoulders and arms will allow.
4 Hold for a count of ten, return to the starting position and repeat the exercise five times.

Fingers on Shoulders

PURPOSE

Expands and opens up chest.
Stretches upper-back and shoulder muscles.

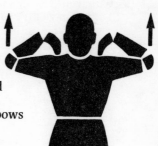

METHOD

1 Stand tall or sit upright.
2 Place the fingertips of both hands on your
  shoulders, keeping your shoulders down,
  level and relaxed.
3 Move your elbows round in large circles.
4 Try to touch your elbows in front, then move them
  in as big a circle as possible round and behind until
  you get back to the starting position.
5 Breathe in as you open up and out as you close
  forward.
6 Repeat the exercise ten times.

Fingers on Shoulders Variation 1

METHOD

1 Raise fingertips to shoulders as before.
2 Keeping fingertips there, raise one elbow up and
  out and lower it towards the floor.
3 Repeat with the other elbow, then with both elbows
  together.
4 Stretch them as high as you can with ease.
5 Repeat the exercise ten times.

POINTS TO NOTE

1 Keep all your movements smooth and gentle.
2 *Do not overstretch or strain.*

75

Fingers on Shoulders Variation 2

METHOD

1 Place your fingertips on your shoulders as before.
2 Keep your elbows in front of your chest.
3 Swing your right elbow as far as possible to the left across your chest. Feel the stretch across your back, chest and shoulders.
4 Repeat with the other elbow, then try to hold both elbows together in front of your chest, then release.
5 Relax and repeat exercise.
6 Repeat the exercise five times.

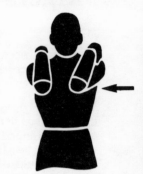

Fingers on Shoulders Variation 3

METHOD

1 Adopt the same position with your fingertips on your shoulders.
2 Swing your elbows out to face away from you, in one plane with your body.
3 As you do this, inhale deeply and lift both elbows and arms upward, still keeping your fingertips on your shoulders.
4 Repeat the exercise five times.

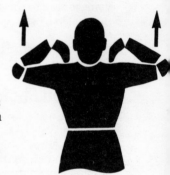

POINTS TO NOTE

1 Keep all your movements smooth and gentle.
2 *Do not overstretch or strain.*

Wrist Rotations

PURPOSE

Loosens up wrists and shoulders.

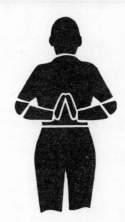

METHOD

1 Stand upright with a good posture and pelvic tilt.
2 Place your hands behind your back with your fingers pointing down towards the floor and your hands open.
3 Simply rotate your wrists so that your fingertips now point up towards the ceiling.
4 Press your palms together if you can. *Do not force.*
5 Hold for a count of twenty, then relax.
6 Repeat the exercise twice.

Palm Press

PURPOSE

Good for chest muscles.

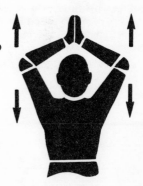

METHOD

1 Stand with a good posture and pelvic tilt and keep your shoulders relaxed. In fact, relax all over.
2 With palms facing, place fingers together, level with chest.
3 Press hands together with short, sharp pushes.
4 Repeat these pushes with your hands overhead and fingers pointing towards the ceiling.
5 Repeat with hands at waist-level, pointing fingers down towards the floor.
6 Repeat each exercise five times.

POINTS TO NOTE

1 *Do not force any of these exercises.*
2 Take things easy at all times.

Hands Behind Neck I

PURPOSE

Stretches shoulders and chest.
Superb exercises for posture improvement.

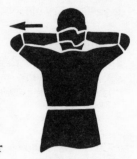

METHOD

1 Either stand or sit.
2 Interlock fingers behind your head at the base of your neck and slowly pull your right arm with your left as far as you can go with ease.
3 Hold for a slow count of ten.
4 Relax and repeat with the other side, pulling your left arm with your right.
5 Repeat the exercise with each arm five times.

Hands Behind Neck I Variation

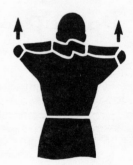

METHOD

1 Either stand or sit.
2 Clasp hands behind neck as before.
3 This time, pull your elbows up and back as if trying to touch the ceiling with the points of your elbows. Raise your elbows as high as you can.
4 Hold for a count of five.
5 Relax and repeat exercise five times.

POINTS TO NOTE

1 Keep your head up with your chin in and a good pelvic tilt.
2 Breathe easily at all times.
3 Try to keep your elbows along the same plane as the rest of your trunk.
4 *Do not sway backward or forward.*

Arms Behind Back

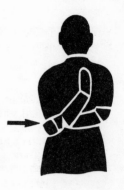

PURPOSE

Loosens up shoulders, helps posture and circulation.

METHOD

1 Stand with a good posture.
2 Bend your left arm at the elbow and take it round behind your back and up between your shoulder-blades, if you can.
3 Try to grasp your left elbow behind your back with your right hand and ease the elbow across towards your right side gently to increase the stretch.
4 Repeat five times.
5 Change arms and repeat the exercise.

Arms Behind Back Variation

METHOD

1 Stand upright with a good posture.
2 Place your hands behind your back with fingers pointing down towards the floor.
3 Grasp your right wrist with your left hand and pull your right arm down and across your back.
4 Hold for a count of ten.
5 Relax, then change arms and repeat.
6 To increase the stretch, tilt your head towards the side of the hand that is pulling down. You will feel the difference in the stretch at once.

POINTS TO NOTE

1 If you cannot reach your elbow behind you, grasp your wrist instead. You will be amazed how soon you will be able to reach your elbow as your muscles loosen up when you practise the stretch.
2 Do what you can to start with and take things easy at all times.

Finger Locks

PURPOSE
Loosens up shoulder muscles and opens up chest.
Stretches triceps and upper-back muscles.

METHOD
1 Stand tall with a good posture, relax shoulders.
2 Take your left hand up and over your left
   shoulder.
3 Reach down as far as you can and try and touch
   your right hand coming up from the other side. Try
   to lock the fingers of both hands together. Many of
   you will be unable to do this as your shoulder
   muscles will be too tight. If you cannot do this:
4 Take a short towel or strap and hold one end in
   your left hand and take that hand up and over
   your left shoulder as before, then your other
   hand can reach the other end of the towel.
5 Gradually try to work your fingers closer together
   and eventually touch. You may find a large gap
   between your hands at first, but persevere.
6 Change arms and repeat. You will almost certainly
   find one side easier than the other which will show
   you immediately where you have shortened
   muscles.
7 Once you have managed to link hands, take the
   top elbow back and down and lower elbow back
   and up as you straighten. Reach down as far as
   you can with the top hand.
8 Hold for a count of ten, change hands and repeat.

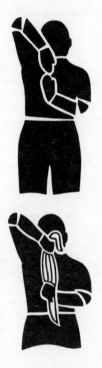

POINTS TO NOTE
1 *Do not overstretch.* Take things easily and gently at all times.
2 Keep your head up, your chin in and your shoulders relaxed.
3 Breathe easily. *You should not feel you are straining anything.*
4 Regular practice will soon have your hands meeting.
5 A marvellous stretch to do at any time, anywhere, especially if you
   are desk-bound.

Arm Pulls

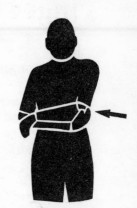

PURPOSE

Loosens shoulders and stretches upper back.

METHOD

1 Stand tall with a good posture.
2 Grasp one elbow with the other hand.
3 Gently pull the elbow across your chest towards the opposite shoulder.
4 Hold for a count of ten.
5 Change arms and repeat the exercise.

Arm Pulls Variation

METHOD

1 Stand tall with a good posture and pelvic tilt.
2 Hold one arm just above the elbow.
3 Gently pull that arm across to the opposite side so that your hand actually goes over your shoulder.
4 Hold for a count of ten then change arms and repeat.
5 When you find this stretch too easy, allow the elbow to push back against the hand grip.

POINTS TO NOTE

1 Keep spine long, stand tall and keep a good pelvic tilt.
2 Keep shoulders relaxed and down.
3 *Do not overstretch.*
4 Always apply an even pressure and take things gently.

Chair Dips

PURPOSE

To strengthen shoulders and arms to ease general
tasks.
Marvellous exercises for building upper-body strength
in the chest and the arms.

METHOD

1 Place your hands on a sturdy chair seat with your
feet on the floor.
2 Keep feet away from the chair to make sure that
your arms do the work.
3 Stretch your legs out and away from the chair so
that your body weight is taken by your arms
resting on the chair seat.
4 Bend your arms and lower your body towards the
ground.
5 Push back to the starting position.
6 Repeat until your arms tire. Start off with just one
or two of these dips at a time until you build up
enough strength to increase the amount; you could
do them in the course of your working day.

POINTS TO NOTE

1 *Do not let your trunk collapse into a jackknife shape.*
2 *Take extra care if you are weak in the arms and shoulders.*
3 Keep your head up and take things gently at all times.
4 Build the exercises up over a period of time.

Arms Overhead

PURPOSE

To stretch shoulders and arms.

METHOD

1 Stand tall with a good posture and pelvic tilt.
2 Keep your knees flexed.
3 Clasp hands together and extend them overhead.
4 Reach up as far as you can, but keep your feet flat on the floor. Feel yourself growing upward.
5 To stretch your sides at the same time, lean gently to each side when your hands are overhead.
6 To help your shoulders and upper arms and release tension, cross palms and wrists together when your arms are overhead, breathe in and stretch upward.
7 Repeat ten times.

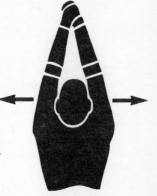

Arms Overhead Variation

METHOD

1 Stand as before.
2 Lace your fingers together and push your palms out and away from you in front at shoulder-level until your arms are straight.
3 Take your arms overhead with your fingers still interlocked and your palms facing the ceiling.
4 Keep elbows, shoulders and back in a straight line.
5 Bend your elbows and allow your hands to come down behind your neck, palms facing your neck.
6 Push them up towards the ceiling again and out to the front then back and relax. Repeat five times.
7 Vary the positions as you feel the benefit.

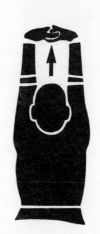

> **POINTS TO NOTE**
> Superb all-round stretches which straighten you up as your shoulders relax and your chest expands.

Triceps Stretch

PURPOSE

Strengthens the back of the upper arms and shoulders and opens up the chest.

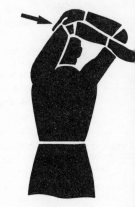

METHOD

1 Stand with a good posture and pelvic tilt.
2 Bend your knees slightly and raise both arms.
3 Curve your right hand and elbow over and behind your head.
4 Bend the left elbow and gently pull it with your right hand, creating a downward stretch.
5 Repeat using the left arm.
6 Repeat the exercise two to five times.

Triceps Stretch Variation

METHOD

1 Stand in the same position as above, knees slightly bent, arms raised.
2 Placing your right hand on your left elbow, pull your raised left arm across towards the other side. Gently pull the elbow but do not bend the left arm.
3 Pull sideways, not downward as in the previous stretch. You will feel the stretch down the side.
4 Hold for a slow count of ten.
5 Repeat, raising the right arm.
6 Repeat each exercise two to five times.
7 You can vary the line of the pull from across to downward as you vary from a straight to a bent elbow. To increase the stretch, bend towards the side of the arm being stretched.

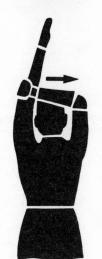

POINTS TO NOTE

Do these exercises slowly and gently.

Neck Turns and Stretches

PURPOSE
Ensures neck flexibility and reduces neck stiffness.

METHOD

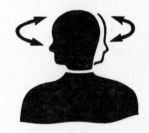

1 Look over one shoulder, then swing your head down and around in a half-circle to look over the other shoulder.
2 To vary this exercise, look over one shoulder then the other, keeping your chin level with the floor. Relax, then try to look a bit further over your shoulder. This will become easier as you practise the exercise. Try to look as far over your shoulder as you can. Keep shoulders down and aim your chin over your shoulder.
3 NEVER drop your head away behind you.
4 Keeping your shoulders facing forward, repeat the exercise ten times.

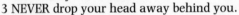

Head Drop I

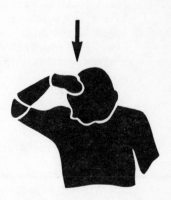

METHOD

1 Stand or sit with a good posture and pelvic tilt.
2 Turn your head to look diagonally (halfway round to the side).
3 Tilt your head and bring it into your chest.
4 Breathe easily throughout.
5 You can vary the stretch by placing your hand on top of your head and pulling down gently.

POINTS TO NOTE

Regular exercise will ensure neck flexibility and reduce neck stiffness which is often the forerunner of neck pains and headaches. Avoid large neck rolls as this can lead to compression of the joints and increased wear and tear. Although the neck is intrinsically strong, never jerk or pull it while exercising.

Neck Pushes

PURPOSE

To strengthen neck muscles and ease neck tension.

METHOD

1 Place your right hand over your right ear.
2 Slowly push your head towards your left shoulder.
3 Try to keep both shoulders level and avoid bringing your left shoulder up to meet your head.
4 Repeat, then change hands and push your head towards your right shoulder.

Neck Pushes Variation

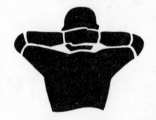

METHOD

1 Place both hands behind your head at neck level.
2 Lock your fingers together.
3 Push back with your head and push your hands against your head.
4 Hold for a count of ten, then relax.
5 Repeat exercise.

POINTS TO NOTE

1 This is a good way of controlling neck exercise.
2 *Do not push too hard.* Push just enough to cause muscles to work.
3 *Do not reach the quivering stage.*
4 Push hard enough to be just short of movement.

Hands Behind Neck II

PURPOSE

Wonderful for easing neck strains.

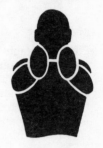

METHOD

1 Place both hands behind your neck and clasp your fingers together.
2 Keeping your fingers laced together, gently pull your elbows forward until they touch in front.
3 Gently push your neck backward against your laced hands.
4 Regain the starting position. Repeat ten times.

Head Drop II

PURPOSE

Eases neck strain and tension.

METHOD

1 Drop your head forward and let it rest as near to your chest as you can easily reach.
2 Lace your fingers behind your neck as above.
3 Allow your elbows to point towards the floor.
4 Using your hands, gently but firmly, pull your head down on to your chest.
5 Hold for a count of ten, then relax.
6 Return to the start and repeat the exercise.
7 You can easily vary this stretch by turning your head very slightly first to one side then the other.

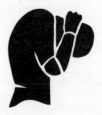

POINTS TO NOTE

1 This is a good way of controlling neck exercise.
2 *Do not push too hard*: hard enough to be just short of movement.
3 *Do not reach the quivering stage*.
4 Keep a good pelvic tilt.

Weight on Head

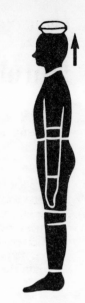

PURPOSE

Helps develop the idea of proper posture.

METHOD

1 Use a suitable book or cushion or better still a bag of flour or sugar weighing no more than two to five pounds (900 g–2·15 kg).
2 Walk, sit or stand erect, with good alignment.
3 Keep your chin in and level.
4 Push your head up into the weight. Try to feel as if you are pushing the weight towards the ceiling.
5 Keep your shoulders down.

Head Slides

PURPOSE

To free neck tension and aid posture.

METHOD

1 Keep your chin level and push your head upward so that the chin comes in and down, then slide your chin back and forth on same plane as if sliding it along a greasy surface.
2 Bring the chin back as far as you can and hold the retracted position longer.
3 Turn your head very slightly to one side and repeat.
4 Repeat as often as you can through the day and you will soon feel the difference.

POINTS TO NOTE

1 The neck is a very common site of pain and responds well to exercise done correctly.
2 Your head position is crucial. Try to keep your back long so that your head is positioned above your shoulders, not in front of them.

Forehead Pushes

PURPOSE

To strengthen the neck muscles and ease neck tension.

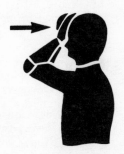

METHOD

1 Place both hands on your forehead, one hand over the other.
2 Push forward with your head and at the same time push your hands back against your head.
3 Hold for a count of ten.
4 Relax, then repeat the exercise.

Forehead Pushes Variation

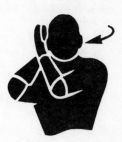

METHOD

1 Place both hands on the right side of the forehead.
2 Attempt to turn your head right while resisting the turn with hand pressure.
3 Hold for a count of ten, then relax.
4 Change sides and turn to the left.

POINTS TO NOTE

1 This is a good way of controlling neck exercise.
2 *Do not push too hard.* Push just enough to cause the muscles to work.
3 *Do not reach the quivering stage.*
4 Push hard enough to be just short of movement.

Neck Potpourri

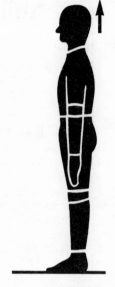

PURPOSE

To encourage better posture and ease neck pain.

Retraction

METHOD

1 Look straight ahead and pull your chin back into a straight, level position.
2 Push the top of your head towards the ceiling, thereby lengthening the distance between your ears and shoulders.
3 You can raise and lower your shoulders slightly to relax them.
4 Feel yourself growing taller each time you do the exercise.

Flexion, Extension, Rotation

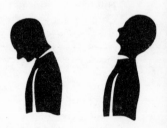

METHOD FOR FLEXION

Tuck your chin in and bend your head forward, keeping shoulders relaxed. Repeat the exercise.

METHOD FOR EXTENSION

Tip your head back as if you were looking at the ceiling, but no further. Repeat exercise.

METHOD FOR ROTATION

Turn your head to look over one shoulder, then slowly turn your head round to look over the other shoulder. Tuck your chin into your chest, keeping your shoulders down and level. Pull shoulders down to increase the effect. Complete head circles are unnecessary.

Leg Swings

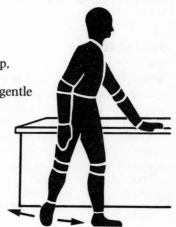

PURPOSE

To loosen up legs and stretch hips.
Helps circulation and tones up thighs.

METHOD

1 Stand sideways to a chair back or worktop,
  resting on one hand for support.
2 Swing your outside leg back and forth in gentle
  arcs of not more than forty-five degrees.
3 Hold a good posture and pelvic tilt.
4 Repeat the exercise ten times.
5 Turn around and repeat the exercise
  with the other leg.
6 Try to keep the exercising leg straight,
  with the stationary leg flexed at the
  knee.

Leg Swings Variation

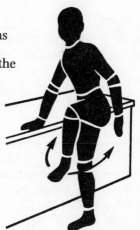

METHOD

1 Hold the chair back or worktop with one hand as
  before.
2 Raise the outer knee up to a right angle so that the
  thigh is parallel to the ground.
3 Gently swing the knee in towards the chair and
  then out in a hundred-and-eighty-degree arc.
4 Repeat five times.
5 Turn around and repeat the exercise with the
  other leg.

POINTS TO NOTE
Take things easily at all times. Do not force anything.

91

Half Squats

PURPOSE

To strengthen the thighs; essential for walking and
correct lifting and bending.
To help back muscles.

METHOD

1 Grasp the chair back or worktop with both hands,
  keeping a good posture and pelvic tilt.
2 Keep feet slightly apart and about eighteen inches
  from the base of the chair or worktop.
3 Slowly bend your knees, keeping your back
  straight.
4 Do not bend too far. Never reach a position where
  your knees are at right angles.
5 Stand upright again using your thigh muscles.
6 Repeat the exercise to suit you.

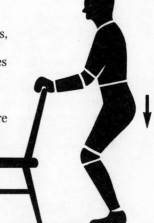

POINTS TO NOTE

1 Do not bend the knees too far. Take things very gently. Do not go
  into a deep squat as this is too much to begin with.
2 Keep your shoulders relaxed and heels down on the floor, with feet
  slightly turned out to aid balance.
3 You will soon notice the difference as your thigh muscles get
  stronger. Adjust the distance from the chair back or worktop to
  vary the amount of stretch.

Most of you will find this exercise difficult in the beginning. It may
help you to rise up on your toes first. Persevere as this is a superb
all-round stretching exercise. Take things slowly. You may manage
only one or two squats at first. Try to work up to ten or twelve
repetitions as your muscles get stronger.
  Do not bend too deep. Keep your back straight with good balance
and control. Your thighs provide the power.

Counter Sink Dips

PURPOSE

To stretch upper back and spine and release tension.
Eases lower back and hamstrings. Marvellous for
round shoulders. A superb all-round stretch.

METHOD

1 Stand about an arm's-length away from a solid
  worktop (you may find a window-sill easier at
  first).
2 Bend your knees, lean forward, fold your arms on
  the surface and rest your head on your folded
  arms.
3 Slowly straighten your knees and feel your spine
  gradually stretch. Keep knees slightly bent.
4 Push your bottom out away from the top
  of your body to increase the stretch,
  but keep a pelvic tilt.

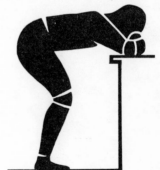

POINTS TO NOTE

1 Keep your shoulders relaxed and use your hands as a balance and
  support.
2 Keep thighs and legs relaxed. Keep a pelvic tilt and look down at
  the floor.
3 Do not arch your back or your neck. Always keep knees slightly
  relaxed to protect your hamstrings.
4 Gently vary the stretch by rounding your back upward then
  flattening it or by rolling your hips, i.e. walking on the spot while
  supporting yourself against the worktop.

Counter Sink Dips Variation

METHOD

1 Try to progress to placing just your hands on the
   worktop.
2 Move further back and once again gently straighten
   your knees and push your buttocks away from the
   worktop.
3 Try to keep your back as straight as possible.
4 Make sure you bend at the hips. Keep knees directly
   under hips.
5 Try to think of lengthening the spine away from
   the worktop, keeping it horizontal.
6 Breathe easily, relax into the stretch and feel
   tension dissipate.

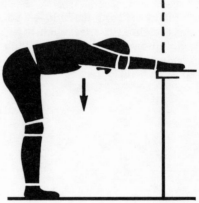

Quadriceps Stretch

PURPOSE

To stretch and strengthen the quadriceps muscles.
To help posture and strengthen the thighs and knees.

METHOD

1 Stand tall with a good posture and pelvic tilt.
2 Hold the chair back or worktop for support with right hand and use the left hand to grasp the left foot and raise it up behind your body towards the left buttock.
3 Gently pull your foot.
4 Hold for a slow count of ten, feeling the stretch down the front of the left thigh.
5 Change legs, hold your right foot and repeat the exercise.
6 Repeat exercise five times with each foot.

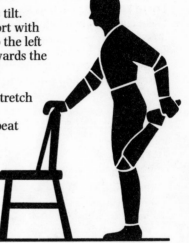

POINTS TO NOTE

1 Keep your shoulders level and spine long with a pelvic tilt.
2 *Do not bend forward.*
3 *Do not bend knee too far.* Use the foot to pull down against your hand to increase the stretch. Pull slowly and evenly, feeling the stretch down the front of the thigh.
4 There is no need for your foot actually to touch your buttock as this overextends the knee-joint.
5 Hold either foot or ankle (whichever suits you best) *gently*. Always try to keep your bent knee pointing towards the floor if you can with the straight knee slightly flexed.
6 *Do not arch your back* and keep hips square.
7 Your shoulders should be down and relaxed.
8 Keep thighs parallel if possible.
9 There should be no jerkiness with this exercise.

95

Groin Hip Stretch

PURPOSE
Helps the lower-back and inner-thigh muscles.

METHOD
1 Sit on the floor, place the soles of your feet together and pull them in towards your body as far as you can without forcing.
2 Slowly and gently, push your knees to the floor using your hands and forearms on your knees.
3 Hold for a count of ten.
4 Release, relax and repeat the exercise.

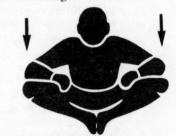

Groin Hip Stretch Variation

METHOD
1 Sit on the floor, place the soles of your feet together and pull them in towards your body as far as you can without forcing.
2 Place one hand on each ankle and gently press your knees to the floor using your elbows.
3 Hold for a count of ten.
4 Release, relax and repeat from the start.
5 As this gets easier, press down a bit more to increase the stretch.
6 Always sit well with relaxed shoulders, a good posture and pelvic tilt.
7 Keep your knees as far out to either side as possible to aid the stretch: let your knees fall to the floor.
8 The secret is to work your knees down gently as your muscles gradually relax. As you feel the tension leave, add a bit more stretch. Hold the position, let the tension go, then stretch again.

POINTS TO NOTE
1 Bend forward very slightly during the exercise to ease the strain on your lower back and breathe easily.
2 Let your legs drop towards the floor, *do not force them.*

Knee to Chest II

PURPOSE

Lengthens hip flexors and helps lower back.

METHOD

1 Lie on your back with both knees up at about forty-five degrees, your feet flat on the floor.
2 Do a pelvic tilt, i.e. flatten your lower back against the floor.
3 Grasp your right leg behind the knee and bring it up to your chest.
4 Hold for a slow count of ten.
5 Release and repeat with your left leg.
6 Repeat five times with each leg.

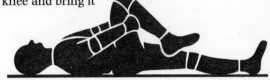

Knee to Chest II Variations

METHOD

1 After doing the above exercise with each leg in turn, repeat lifting both knees to your chest at the same time.
2 Lift your head gently off the floor to touch your knees if you can. Your buttocks will come off the floor as your lower back stretches.
3 To vary this, once you have got both your knees up to your chest, rock gently back and forth.
4 When you have got used to these exercises, try raising one knee to your chest, then stretching the other leg out flat on the floor. You can also try pointing the raised leg straight towards the ceiling, stretching the groin as well as the hip, *but do not raise both legs off the floor at the same time or try to force anything.*

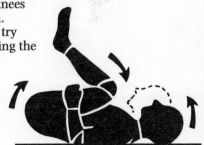

POINTS TO NOTE

1 Use *both* hands clasped behind your knees to raise your legs to your chest and pull gently. *Do not jerk your knees.*
2 Keep a good pelvic tilt. *Do not let your back arch off the floor.*
3 Always lower yourself slowly and gently back down.

97

Curl Ups

PURPOSE

Strengthens abdominal muscles.

METHOD

1 Lie flat on the floor with your knees bent at forty-five degrees.
2 Stretch your arms out alongside you.
3 Breathe in and curl your neck and upper back up a little, but no more than forty degrees, as you breathe out.
4 Try to touch your fingers to your knees and eventually to slide your hands up to your knees.
5 Hold for five seconds.
6 Lower yourself slowly and repeat ten times if you can.

Curl Ups Variation

METHOD

1 Lie on the floor, keeping your lower back flat with a good pelvic tilt.
2 Twist very slightly as you curl forward. Your abdominal muscles are used most in the first few inches therefore it is unnecessary to come up too far. *Do not go past forty degrees.*
3 Curl your head before you curl your neck.
4 Progress to curling upwards with your arms folded across your chest, to a forty-degree angle, no more.
5 Hold for five seconds then repeat.

POINTS TO NOTE

1 Keep your lower back flat on the floor with a good pelvic tilt.
2 There is no advantage to be gained by coming up past forty degrees as, after this, your hips and back muscles will take over which can lead to back problems and is also a waste of energy. Just let your shoulders come off the floor.
3 Curl back slowly to the floor.
4 You can progress from having your arms at your sides to putting your arms behind your head with your elbows to the sides.
5 *Do not jerk upwards.* Do these exercises slowly and carefully.

Sit Backs

PURPOSE

Strengthens back and abdominal muscles.

METHOD

1 Sit on the floor with your knees bent to about forty-five degrees. It is best *not* to anchor your feet to do this exercise.
2 Put your hands behind your head with your elbows out to the sides and lean back slowly until you feel a mild strain.
3 Breathe out slowly as you curl back.
4 Hold for a count of five and feel your tummy muscles working.
5 Return to the starting position.
6 Repeat as often as you can with ease. You may only be able to do one or two of these at first, but more as you get stronger.
7 To make it easier for you in the beginning, start off by holding your knees as you sit back. Relax the grip on your knees as you get stronger.
8 As a variation of the above exercise, keep your hands straight out in front of you at shoulder-level instead of putting them behind your head before you lean slowly back.

POINTS TO NOTE

1 Just go back forty-five degrees to start with, no further. As you get stronger, you can go back further. You will know when the time comes. These exercises all help to strengthen your abdominal muscles and help you keep a good pelvic tilt. Weak abdominal muscles are a common cause of back ache and poor posture.
2 Do these exercises *very slowly*. The benefit lies in slow and controlled movement.
3 Keep the lower back straight with a good pelvic tilt.
4 *Remember, do not force movement at any time.*

Floor Potpourri

PURPOSE

Exercises to strengthen shoulder, arm and upper-back muscles. Ideal for rest, relaxation and warm-ups.

Spinal Rock and Roll

METHOD

1 Lie on the floor.
2 Hold both legs behind the knees and bring them up to your chest.
3 Bring your forehead up gently to touch your knees if you can reach without straining.
4 Hold this position and gently rock back and forth along your spine to massage the vertebrae.
5 Keep completely relaxed as you rock.
6 Be sure to keep the swings small and gentle – feel your back relax.

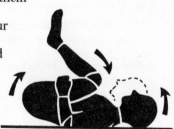

Alexander Technique Relaxation

METHOD

1 Lie down flat with your arms at your sides and your legs stretched out.
2 Keep a good pelvic tilt.
3 Bend your knees towards the ceiling at forty-five degrees with your feet flat on the floor.
4 Place one or two books under your head to support your neck. You will have to experiment with the number of books required to ensure your head is kept level, i.e. not pulling back too much or pushing forward thereby causing your chin to be pushed down on your chest which will constrict your throat. Some people need more books to support their head than others.
5 Keep your chin pointing towards the ceiling.
6 Lie in this position and totally relax.

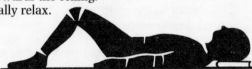

Ten Exercises That are Especially Helpful for Back Protection

These exercises will help to lay a solid foundation for the care and defence of your back and should be done regularly.

Exercises That Can be Done at Any Time, Anywhere

Exercises 4 and 5 are best done at home.

Strength Exercises

Here are a few suggested combinations of standing exercises – both for a free-standing position and using a wall or door.

Combination 1

1 Wall Squats   54
2 Side Bends   43
3 Trunk Twists   46
4 Slumps   47

Combination 2

1 Chest Stretches I   59
2 Chest Arm Flings   50
3 Wall Squats   54
4 Side Bends   43

Combination 3

1 Wall Stand   56
2 Wall Turns   62
3 Side Bends   43
4 Wood Chopper   50

Combination 4

1 Wall Stand   56
2 Hip Circles   44
3 Chest Stretches I   59
   Variation 2   60
4 Ceiling Reaches   42

Combination 5

1 Knee to Chest I   61
2 Side Bends to Wall   53
3 Hip Circles   44
4 Slumps   47

Combination 6

1 Tendon Stretches   58
2 Finger Wall Walk   61
3 Trunk Twists   46
4 Wall Turns   62

Combination 7

1 Wall Stand   56
2 Wall Squats   54
3 Chest Stretches I   59
4 Side Bends   43

Combination 8

1 Tendon Stretches   58
2 Half Knee Bends   45
3 Hamstring Stretch   51
4 Knee to Chest I   61

Here are a few seated combinations involving the shoulder and arm exercises as well as the neck exercises.

Combination 1

1 Chest Stretches II   65
2 Head Drop I   85
3 Arm Pulls   81
4 Seated Breathing   64

Combination 2

1 Body Hugs   64
2 Laced Finger Stretch   70
3 Neck Pushes   86
4 Fingers on Shoulders   75

Combination 3

1 Chair Slumps   67
2 Chair Dips   82
3 Forehead Pushes   89
4 Hands Behind Neck II   87

Combination 4

1 Calf Stretch   63
2 Hands Behind Back   73
3 Chest Arm Pull   66
4 Neck Turns   69

Combination 5

1 Pelvic Slides   68
2 Chair Slumps   67
3 Neck Pushes   86
4 Arms Overhead   83

Combination 6

1 Chest Stretches I   59
2 Laced Finger Stretch   70
3 Head Drop II   87
4 Fingers on Shoulders   75

Combination 7

1 Forehead Pushes   89
2 Fingers on Shoulders   75
3 Wrist Rotations   77
4 Laced Finger Stretch   70

Combination 8

1 Hands Behind Neck I   78
2 Head Drop I   85
3 Palm Press   77
4 Arm Pulls   81

Combination 9

1 Hands Behind Back   73
2 Fingers on Shoulders   75
3 Neck Turns and Stretches   85
4 Triceps Stretch   84

Combination 10

1 Arms Overhead   83
2 Head Drop I   85
3 Finger Locks   80
4 Neck Pushes   86

Combination 11

1 Neck Turns 69
2 Arms Overhead 83
3 Chair Dips 82
4 Hands Behind Neck II 87

Combination 12

1 Ankle Circles 63
2 Chair Slumps 67
3 Forehead Pushes 89
4 Neck Turns 69

These combinations are only suggestions and you can use any of the variations given for each exercise to suit yourself. Remember, there is no compulsion about any of these exercise routines, but a mixture of, say, two sets of the standing combinations plus two sets of the seated combinations will give you a workout that won't take long. It will get easier as you become familiar with the exercises themselves and find out which ones you like to do regularly. Many of the shoulder, arm and neck exercises can be performed in either a standing or sitting position. They have been grouped this way to make it easier to pick them out but do them as you wish.

The following exercises may be done whenever you choose and have been designed to fit easily into your normal day.

Worktop

Floor Exercises

These are obviously easier to do at home but should be done regularly if possible as they will reinforce the flexibility you are developing.

Learn to relax with your head resting on a book (or books) as described on page 100.

We hope that you will come to enjoy doing these exercises knowing that you are accepting the need to protect your back. No one can help you as well as you can help yourself.

Further Reading

The following books could be useful for further information on various aspects of back care, and provide wider knowledge to enhance your exercise regime:

Richard Brennan, *The Alexander Technique Workbook*, Element Books, 1992. (This book and Jonathan Drake's book on the Alexander technique delve more fully into body use and abuse.)

Dr Anthony Campbell, *Getting the Best for your Bad Back*, Sheldon Press, 1992.

Dr Vernon Coleman, *How to Conquer Backache*, Hamlyn, 1993.

Scott Donkin, *Fit for Work*, Kogan Page, 1990.

Jonathan Drake, *Body Know-How*, Thorsons, 1991.

Dr David Imrie with Colleen Dimson, *Goodbye Backache*, Sheldon Press, 1989.

Sarah Keys, *Back in Action*, Random Century, 1991; and *Body in Action*, BBC Books, 1992.

Jenny Sutcliffe, *The Complete Book of Relaxation Techniques*, Headline, 1993. (This book introduces many relaxation techniques to back up the exercise programme.)

The exercises shown in this book are also available in sets of A5 cards. The sets, supplied in folders, may be purchased either individually, for personal use, or in bulk, for use in office or factory.

Please contact:
Dunkeld Publishing
PO Box 2153,
Bournemouth, BH3 7YP.

or telephone 0202 532095 for further information.